How To Feel Great At Work Every Day

Other Books And Programs By Deborah Brown-Volkman

Books Written By Deborah Brown-Volkman:

- *Coach Yourself To A New Career: A Guide For Discovering Your Ultimate Profession*
- *Four Steps To Building A Profitable Coaching Practice: A Complete Marketing Resource Guide For Coaches*
- *Four Steps To Building A Profitable Business: A Marketing Start-Up Guide For Business Owners, Entrepreneurs, And Professionals*

Books Deborah Brown-Volkman Has Contributed To:

- *Essential Coaching Book: Secrets To A Winning Life From The Professional And Personal Coaches Of The United Coaching Associates, Inc.*
- *The Business And Practice Of Coaching*
- *101 Great Ways To Improve Your Life*

Programs Created By Deborah Brown-Volkman:

- *Career Escape Program (Discover Your Dream Job In 4 Weeks)*
- *What To Say When (Techniques To Ask For {And Get}) What You Want In Your Career)*
- *Eight-Step Seminar Series That Walks You Through Finding Your Ultimate Profession*
- *Two-Part Teleclass Series That Walks You Through Building A Profitable Coaching Practice*

- *Three-Part Coaching Seminar Series That Walks You Through Becoming A Full-Time Coach*
- *Coaching Career Transitions (How To Become A Successful Career Coach)*
- *90-Day Teleclass Program To Get Your Name In Print And Gain Worldwide Media Exposure*

All books and programs can be found on Deborah Brown-Volkman's web site at http://www.surpassyourdreams.com

How To Feel Great At Work Every Day

Six Steps For Creating A High-Energy Success Plan For Your Career

Deborah Brown-Volkman
Author of *Coach Yourself To A New Career*

iUniverse, Inc.
New York Lincoln Shanghai

How To Feel Great At Work Every Day
Six Steps For Creating A High-Energy Success Plan For Your Career

iUniverse books may be ordered through booksellers or by contacting:

iUniverse
2021 Pine Lake Road, Suite 100
Lincoln, NE 68512
www.iuniverse.com
1-800-Authors (1-800-288-4677)

ISBN-13: 978-0-595-41263-1 (pbk)
ISBN-13: 978-0-595-85617-6 (ebk)
ISBN-10: 0-595-41263-7 (pbk)
ISBN-10: 0-595-85617-9 (ebk)

Printed in the United States of America

Contents

Acknowledgements

I would like to thank my husband, Brian Volkman, who continues to amaze me with his love, support, and kindness.

I would like to thank the experts in this book who have touched my life and changed the way I look and feel. I admire their positive outlook and commitment to health, energy, and vitality.

I would like to thank the Moriches Beanery for giving me a place to sit and write while drinking the best iced tea that I have ever had in my life.

I would like to acknowledge you, the reader, for realizing that it's time to bring more energy into your career and for having the courage to pick up this book and read it.

Testimonials From Previous Books

"I read your book and loved it. It is an excellent book. I am sure the feedback from your readers has already indicated this." Gale Weithers, Ernst & Young

"I just downloaded your book and I have been unable to put it down. I've been working on the exercises, and all I can say is thank you. I have been very unhappy with my work for quite some time now, and going through your book has made me realize that I am in control, and my choices are up to me." Jodie Thomas, Senior Consultant, Human Resource Management Services

"I have just read your book. It is probably the single best business book I have ever read. It is clear and informative, and there is real value on every page." Corry Robertson

"This is a great book with a lot of valuable information." Sandy Vilas, Master Certified Coach and CEO, CoachInc.com

"This is a great book—thorough, professional, and easy to read." Judy Feld, Master Certified Coach and President of the International Coach Federation (ICF) 2003

"I ordered your book from amazon.com about two weeks ago. I picked it up yesterday with the intention of looking it over to decide if I would read it first or choose another book from my pile. I opened your book at 10:00 PM last night and did not put it down until I finished it. I just couldn't stop reading it. I got so many new ideas. Thank you for your book and for all the wonderful information you shared with me." Beverly Mason, Licensed Professional Counselor

"I purchased your book and wanted to let you know that it is an outstanding book and resource. I started reading it today. It has me thinking differently already." La-Dana Renée Jenkins, Founder, LRJ Consulting Services LLC

"The exercises, wisdom, true-life stories, and guidance contained in this amazing book are the light at the end of the tunnel." Susan Eckert, MA, CCM, Principal, Advance Career and Professional Development

"In this book you will find warmth, guidance, support, and applause." Siegmundo Hirsch, PhD, Career Coach and Counselor

"A must-read." ExecuNet, an Executive Job Search company that meets the needs of $100K+ executives and the companies and recruiters who seek to attract them

Introduction

Having energy is crucial to career success. When you are tired, stressed, or burned out, you don't have the motivation to do things beyond what your job responsibilities entail. Sometimes, you might not have the energy to meet even these basic duties. In the workplace, however, how you feel is not important to your employers or clients. You have a job to do, and you have to do it regardless of your mood or energy level.

When you have energy, you can do things in your career that might otherwise be impossible. You gain passion, power, and focus. Procrastination is nonexistent. Your productivity increases. You know what you want, and you feel great about it.

Personal energy is an important key to career advancement. If you want to further your career by going back to school at night, you need energy. If you want a promotion, you may need extra energy to develop a new idea or concept. If you want a great life, you need energy to enjoy the company of your family and friends when you are not working. If you want to lose weight, you need energy to get up early and exercise. Energy has the power to transform your career and your life for the better.

I am no stranger to low energy. Until recently, I had been tired at work for as long as I can remember. Before I became a coach, entrepreneur, and business owner, I ran sales and marketing programs for Fortune 500 and technology companies for over twelve years. I worked a lot. My jobs were in New York City, whose hectic pace demanded a great deal of energy. I was expected to perform at a high level, and adrenaline played an important role in getting many things done.

Then I switched careers. I built a coaching business from scratch, which took a lot of my time and energy. I worked round the clock and gained forty pounds. Even though I was helping people change their careers and their lives (and loving every minute of my job), a part of me knew that I needed to get healthier.

Furthermore, the adrenaline I so depended on to keep me going was beginning to run low.

For most of my career, much of my energy and ability to perform and produce steady work came from processed foods, refined sugar, and caffeine. If I was tired in the morning, caffeine would help me start my day. If I was tired in the afternoon, I would eat chocolate and immediately feel better. If I wanted a pick-me-up at the end of the day, chips or pretzels would give me a buzzing feeling. This system of getting good results from bad sources worked for a while. It seemed that there was always a solution for my tiredness.

But over time, my body began to change. Small things escalated. What started as occasional indigestion became full-blown reflux disease. What started as occasional discomfort when I closed my pants became constant bloatedness that never seemed to disappear. The food I was eating didn't seem to be digesting properly, and I began to dread mealtimes because I felt worn-out after eating. One day, I looked in the mirror and realized that I was heavier than I'd ever been and getting fatter every day. I tried dieting, but diets would no longer work. I was exhausted. My body ached. I felt old. I had no energy and could not figure out what was wrong with me. For a while, I stopped trying to find out because I thought that being tired was a normal part of getting older. But deep down, I knew that there had to be more to my career and life than being tired. Basically, I got tired of being tired. This is when I put myself on a path to better health. I reached out to people who knew more than me—experts who would help me get better. The amazing people who have helped me get my energy back are some of the same experts I will mention in this book, in addition to other great people I have met in the process of writing it. I am grateful for having them in my life.

Today, in my forties, I feel better than I did when I was younger. I have reduced my stress level considerably. I sleep better. I exercise. I eat better foods. I make time to shop for healthier foods because I know that if I don't, I won't feel well. I'm not bloated any more and have lost weight. I feel strong and optimistic. And finally, I have written this book—a project that would have been impossible only a short time ago, because I would have been too tired to do it. Am I perfect? No, But I get up every day with the energy to try my best. I am on a different path now and am happy that I found it.

As a career coach, I speak to hundreds of people each year who are unhappy with their careers. When I ask them what they eat, how physically active they are, and how they handle stress, their answers do not surprise me. One by one, they tell me that they are not taking care of themselves. No wonder they are unhappy. How can they love what they do when they don't feel their best? How can they build momentum in their careers when they are tired? How can they fulfill their dreams when they don't have the energy to make it happen?

Every day I see what people do to themselves—not eating right, not sleeping enough, not exercising, working too much—without realizing the consequences. I understand that such behavior has become a way of life for many people, but I am saddened that they think that this is the only way to live. I wrote this book to help them.

I wrote this book because I noticed that something was missing from the books that are in the market today. There are plenty of books on how to gain more energy, but not many on how to gain more energy *at work*. I also found books that had great advice for increasing energy; but their suggestions, though helpful, were difficult to follow or understand.

I wrote this book to help you create a practical plan to get more energy for use in your career. This book is not filled with complicated suggestions and ideas. There are no concepts that you have to go back to school to learn. This book gives you immediately useful steps that you can implement in your career, no matter what it happens to be.

Change is possible. You can have more energy, even with your hectic schedule and busy life. No matter what habits you have formed, you can form new ones. No matter what has happened to your energy level, it can be increased. No matter what your age, you can make a difference to your body, mind, and spirit. As with all change, starting will be the hardest part. But over time, your starting point will become a distant memory, and you will find that you have been left with new habits that inspire and empower you. Huge amounts of energy are within your reach, and I will help you take steps in its direction.

Note: I have created a wonderful online resource to assist you, in addition to the book you are reading.

To register to receive *free* access to a special web page that contains further information and steps toward increased energy in your career, please visit:
http://www.surpassyourdreans.com/energyresources.html

Once you register, you will be notified of exclusive groups and classes, which I will be conducting by telephone, about obtaining added energy at work. You will also be informed of important energy updates. I hope you will take advantage of this resource I have created just for you.

How To Use This Book

This book is divided into sections. There are six steps to help you get your energy back that includes a roadmap for creating a high-energy career success plan. There are tips, techniques, and suggestions written by experts to help guide you. There are resources you can continue to use once you have finished reading the book and implementing its concepts. The book is a full package to help you obtain more energy in your career.

The book contains simple and straightforward concepts. I believe that more complicated techniques would serve only to slow your progress. You may read portions of this book and say to yourself, "I know that already." Indeed, for many of you, most of what you need to know you have already learned. But the question you must ask yourself is: "Am I using my knowledge in the best ways I possibly can?" My goal, above all, is to help you use your knowledge effectively.

Once you have created your high-energy career success plan, you will want to see results right away. This is normal. As human beings, once we have set a goal, we want to reach it immediately. We want what we want when we want it. This is our nature. You are reading this book because you want to change. You want to feel better. You want a great career. These are commendable goals.

Change is a journey that happens one step at a time. If you try to implement all six of the steps too quickly, you will become overwhelmed. Feeling overwhelmed is counterproductive. It kills momentum and the desire to succeed. If you try to do too much, you greatly increase your chances of failure.

My advice is that you read one step and then take time to contemplate the information. Make the step and the concepts your own. Only when you feel comfortable with one step should you move on to the next one. Small steps taken over time in this manner will lead you to your high-energy career goal.

Remember that your energy level took time to decline. And so, it will need time to rise. Give yourself the freedom and space to create a plan that you will be able to use for the rest of your life.

Good luck!

Why You Struggle With Low Energy

Being tired and having low energy is likely common in your workplace. How can it not be? You've been getting up early five days or more per week for years. You probably get home late from work, and you go to bed late. Getting eight hours of sleep at night may be a strange concept for you.

You work in a global marketplace. From the moment you arrive at your job, to the moment you leave, you are working. E-mails arrive relentlessly. You may not have control over the work you do, or the people who give it to you. You can work hard on projects that never get implemented and complete projects in days that require weeks to finish properly. You often work more than is good for you because you want money and the luxuries it can buy. But when overworking begins to damage your body and your mind, you may find yourself unable to enjoy all the material things you have worked so hard to obtain.

You keep going even when your body (which knows its limits even when your mind doesn't) wants you to stop. You are oblivious to the warning signs because you don't pause long enough to heed them. Time seems to escape you, and your days become a blur. You might even forget what day it is. You live for the weekends, but two days or less is not long enough to recover and regroup. You realize that this state of affairs can't go on, but how can you change when your time is consumed with work?

You work hard to get ahead, but your extreme focus on your job makes it difficult for you to keep any focus on yourself. You put yourself last. You no longer have boundaries, and yet you feel trapped.

You are tired. Your sleep patterns are off. You feel sluggish during the day, yet you have trouble sleeping at night. You have worked on being successful in your career—going to the right school, wearing the right clothes, having the right network—yet you don't put as much emphasis on your mind and body, which are your two most important tools. You put more effort into planning a vacation than into ensuring that you have enough energy to get through the workday. A vacation lasts for a week or two. How are you planning for the rest of the year?

You know you need to exercise, but you don't. You pack your gym bag in the morning, but it often stays unopened. You say to yourself that you will take a walk at lunch, but then a big project lands on your desk, and you feel that you can't get away from it, even for an hour. You know that you need to reduce your stress levels, but you don't know how. How can you relax your body when you can't even relax your mind?

As your workload and stress levels increase, so does your waistline. When you are hungry, you tend to want something quick, and quick processed foods are too often at your fingertips. You know that "quick" doesn't equal "nutritious," but it makes you feel good and is better than not eating at all. Cookies, doughnuts, desktop candy jars, and other tasty treats surround you. The vending machine containing fast energy boosts is nearby. You skip breakfast, eat sugary junk foods, and drink coffee all day. You binge at night because you are starving or crashing from the chemicals you've put into your body during the day.

Obesity levels are at an all-time high. In *Personnel Today's* exclusive survey of more than 2,000 HR professionals regarding obesity[1], the following facts and figures were cited:

- Twelve percent of people surveyed suggest that obese workers are not suitable for client-facing roles
- Ninety-three percent would employ the 'normal weight' person and only seven percent would employ the obese one
- Thirty percent agree that "obesity is a valid medical reason for not employing a person"
- Forty-seven percent think that obesity negatively affects employee output
- Eleven percent think that employers can fairly dismiss people just because they are obese

A study done by Pfizer Inc. discovered that the obesity rate among American workers of all ages grew from 20 percent to 29 percent over the past decade. The study also found that obese workers are limited in the amount of work they can do; they cannot work as many hours; and they have more mental, physical, and emotional problems.[2]

According to a FOX television-news segment,[3] everyone wants a fat paycheck, but chances are your job is making *you* fat instead. FOX referenced a survey of more than 1,600 workers done by Careerbuilder.com, which showed that 47 percent of Americans had gained weight at their current jobs.

Recent studies, including two from the American Dietetic Association,[4] have shown that more than a third of office workers have breakfast alongside their keyboards, as many as two-thirds regularly munch on lunch in their offices, nine in ten snack on the job, and 7 percent have dinner at their desks. This means that you probably are not taking a proper amount of time to enjoy your food or to give yourself a much-needed break.

Stress, poor eating habits, overwork, and lack of physical activity are key factors that contribute to your tiredness and lethargy during the day. If you are feeling tired, I want you to know that you can win the energy game if you want to, no matter how great the challenges you face.

Use this book to help you win that game.

Step 1:
Recognize That You Have An Energy Problem

Mindy works for a national supermarket chain. Her weight has fluctuated her entire life. When Mindy was young, her parents got divorced. This is when she became secluded and began gaining weight. As Mindy got older, her love of sugar, chocolate, and soda contributed to more weight gain. An inactive, repetitive job in a small office, with candy around her all the time, added more weight. Three pregnancies and late-night ice cream cravings added more.

One day, Mindy went to the doctor. The doctor told Mindy that she had high blood pressure and sent her for a range of tests. He also told Mindy that she was obese. This was her wake-up call.

Mindy went on a fast and lost ten pounds in two weeks. She stopped eating at night and lost another twenty pounds. Mindy was eating healthier and feeling better. Then she injured herself and had to have surgery. She spent six weeks at home recovering and started overeating again.

A year and half later, Mindy was feeling tired and not at all well. She knew that she had to do something about it, so she made a decision to join a weight-loss program. This is when her weight finally started to come down for good. Mindy's weight loss and journey to better health and energy began when she recognized that she had a problem, and she put a plan in place to solve it.

Starting at age thirty-nine, Mindy lost 109 pounds. She lost the weight in eighteen months.

Today, Mindy is a completely different person. She changed jobs and is more active. She exercises daily. Every morning, Mindy has a healthy breakfast consisting of cereal, milk, and fruit. For lunch, she has a cup of yogurt with granola. When Mindy is thirsty, she drinks water instead of soda. When Mindy wants to snack at work, she chews gum or has a piece of fruit, both healthy and inexpensive choices. And perhaps most importantly, she walks past the foods that tempt her.

Initially, Mindy had lost some weight because the doctor had frightened her into it. Now, she keeps the weight off for herself.

DO YOU HAVE A PROBLEM?

Here are some comments I've heard while writing this book and talking to people about feeling great and having more energy to devote to their careers:

"I can't eat better. I'm too busy."

"I can't exercise. I am exhausted when I come home at night."

"I eat the cookies and cake in the kitchen, conference room, or vending machine because they are there."

"I don't like the taste of fruits and vegetables."

"The more work I do, the more tired I get."

High energy is not something that happens by accident. You have to work at it. But what do you do when you don't have the energy to begin? Begin somewhere, with one small step. Begin where you are right now, with as large of a step as you have the energy to take.

You cannot begin to get more energy until you recognize that low energy is a problem for you. Recognition begins with awareness.

Ask yourself the following questions:

- How do I feel in the morning?
- Am I sleeping well?
- Am I eating well?
- Am I making time for physical activity?

- Am I stressed?

- Am I overworked?

- Am I dragging during the day?

And these questions are only the first of many. Others are: What is it costing you to not feel your best every day? Do you come home at night in a bad mood? Do you dread going to work in the morning? Are you not advancing at the pace you'd like? Do you sit at your desk and wonder how you are going to make it through the day? Do you love what you do?

When you are tired, what are you reaching for to give you energy? Sugar? Caffeine? Carbohydrates? How are you handling the highs and lows these choices invariably produce? One moment you may feel great and the next you find yourself irritated and shaky. How does it feel to be a slave to things that keep you going so ineffectively?

How does your body feel? Are you achy? Do you assume that these aches and pains are solely due to your getting older?

Are you agitated? Do you think about your job even when you are not working? Do you wake up in the middle of the night worried about a project that you are responsible for? Do you yawn a lot during the day?

After answering these questions, you may realize that, without your being fully aware of it, your energy level has been declining. Little by little, the food you have been eating, the exercise you have been avoiding, and the stress of your job have been sapping your energy level. Maybe you don't even realize that you have a problem because you have been going at a fast pace for so long and have come to consider it to be "normal." Or maybe you don't believe that you have a choice. After all, you have bills to pay and people counting on you. You have to keep moving in order to survive.

The good news is that low energy is something you can live with for a while. Your body can handle it. The bad news is that one day, your body just won't be able to do it anymore. This is when you will start to encounter larger problems. At first, the problems will be small. You have a cold that won't go away. You have a pain in your back from time to time. Then the problems progress. Your back goes out and you miss a week of work. You get the flu and are in bed for days. Then the problems escalate. You find out you have a cancerous lump. You get a divorce because your stress level took a toll on your marriage. You have reached the point at which you have interfered with your career and your ability to make money and provide for your family.

But there is more good news. You can turn low energy around. Once you become aware and realize what you have been doing, you can put yourself on a path toward understanding how to change it.

WHAT IS SAPPING YOUR ENERGY?

When you are tired at work, you want something that will wake you up fast. You have projects to finish and are under pressure to produce results quickly. It would be nice to take a nap to refresh, but most of us do not have that luxury. So, instead, you reach for something that will wake you up right now. Unfortunately, the things that tend to be available give you "false" energy, meaning that you will feel better for a short time, and then you will crash. When that happens, you will want more of what gave you that brief spurt of energy, so that you can feel better again. You will then crash again and the cycle will continue, to your detriment. It's hard to stop the cycle until you understand the damage that it does to your mind and body.

A High-Energy Disclosure

This section of the book is dedicated to giving you real information about what you are doing to and putting into your body to get more energy. Since I am a career coach, my expertise and training is in the area of helping individuals love their career. I have experienced low energy and found a way out of it. This is why I wrote this book. But still, credentials count, so I will be quoting experts in this section who have written exceptional pieces that will help you understand what you are relying on and doing to give you energy today and how it will hurt you tomorrow. Information is power, and it's important to be informed by people who are outstanding in their fields.

Refined Sugar

Rino Soriano, a Holistic Wellness Consultant & Health Coach and author of *The Chronic Fatigue Buster,* has written an article titled "Sugar Lovers Beware[5]." In this article, Mr. Soriano discusses the effects of refined sugar on our mind and body. Below you will find some important points from his article.

> Refined sugar is one of the worst ingredients to put into your body. The chemical reaction of this type of sugar in the body acts as a poison and has a drug-like effect.
>
> Refined sugar has many harmful effects throughout the body and can cause major imbalances in the organ systems. It tends to throw off the homeostatic balance of the whole body by increasing the production of adrenaline by many times. In essence, refined sugar stimulates the nervous system by inducing a flight-or-fight response. This intense reaction of the body increases the production of cortisone, which suppresses immune function and can lead to other health disorders.
>
> Too much refined sugar intake gives one a false sense of energy. When you eat a sweet food, your energy will go up; however, it only feels that your energy is going up. In fact, this false energy is really your body being stimulated. After this reaction has worn off, your energy levels will come crashing down.

If you have low energy, refined sugar, in the long term, will not give you the energy you are looking for. You will feel better in the moment, but over time you will need more and more of it to get the same feeling, while doing repeated damage to your body.

Caffeine

Emily Clark, an editor at *Lifestyle Health News* and *Medical Health News,*[6] has written an article about the negative effects of caffeine. Here's an excerpt:

> Caffeine is big business. There are new coffee shops popping up all over the place. You can't go far without running into a Starbucks. "Let's get together for coffee. Time for a coffee break. Coffee-pot goes off before your feet hit the floor. Travel mugs for sipping coffee on your way to work. I'll just have this chocolate bar to pick me up this afternoon." Caffeine—it's everywhere.

Many people have grown so accustomed to having their morning coffee or soda that they don't even consider the damaging effects caffeine has on the body. On the contrary, most will tell you that they *need* their jolt to get them moving in the morning or to keep them upright throughout the day. Caffeine is present not only in coffee, but also in tea, soda, chocolate, and in certain pain relievers such as aspirin and acetaminophen. It is also sometimes used in combination with an antihistamine, in order to overcome the drowsiness caused by the antihistamine.

If you don't think it's addicting, try going off caffeine, cold turkey. See if you don't have a headache for two to nine days. That's caffeine withdrawal. You don't need to be a coffeeholic to experience negative physical symptoms. Even as little as one to two cups a day can negatively affect you.

You may be experiencing a number of physical ailments that could be caused solely from caffeine. The most common side effects of caffeine include dizziness, headache, irritability, muscle tension, nausea, nervousness, stuffy nose, unusual tiredness, and jitters.

Too much caffeine can give you all sorts of grief, such as stomach pain, agitation, anxiety, restlessness, confusion, seizures, dehydration, faster breathing rate, fast heartbeat, fever, frequent urination, increased sensitivity to touch or pain, irritability, muscle trembling or twitching, vomiting (sometimes with blood), fibrocystic breast disease, ringing or other sounds in the ears, seeing flashes of zig-zagging lights, and trouble sleeping.

Caffeine may get you going, but after a while, you won't feel its effects as much and will need more of it to keep you going.

Bad Carbohydrates

Hearthstone Communications Ltd. has posted an excellent article on its web site titled "The Real Deal on Carbohydrates."[7] All articles on this web site are written, researched, and published by Monnica Williams. Here are some important points she covers:

Carbohydrates are one of your body's main energy sources. Carbohydrates function as a fuel source for each and every cell in your body. When you eat foods containing carbohydrates, your body breaks down these carbohydrates and converts them into a simple sugar known as glucose. The production of this glucose stimulates your body to produce a hormone known as insulin, which allows your body to transfer the glucose around your body. Any excess glucose is stored in the liver and muscles for future use.

Carbohydrates have been blamed for causing weight gain when eaten in excessive quantities. And unfortunately, this rumor does seem to be based on fact. When you eat carbohydrates, your body breaks them down into glucose to help fuel your cells. Excess glucose is stored in your liver and muscles, but these body parts can only store a certain amount of glucose. Remaining glucose is laid down as fat in certain areas of your body. If you continually ingest large amounts of carbohydrates, it is possible to gain weight.

Some researchers have also linked excessive carbohydrate intake with an increased risk for type-II diabetes. In order to use glucose as fuel, your body needs to produce insulin; therefore, the more glucose your body makes, the more insulin it is required to produce. It appears that some people become overwhelmed by this constant need to supply insulin, and, eventually, become unable to regulate insulin production. This leads to the development of type-II diabetes.

Bad carbohydrates are found in refined foods like cakes, candy, and white bread. These carbs are termed "bad" because they contain little nutritional benefit. Additionally, because they are broken down so quickly in the body, they can actually cause you to feel hungrier faster. Many researchers and health-care experts blame the rising obesity rate in the United States on the increase in bad carbohydrates in our daily diets.

The energy you get from eating bad carbohydrates will only increase your cravings for other refined foods that lack nutritional benefits. Any happiness you feel will be fleeting. There is nothing wrong with carbohydrates as described in this article every once in a while, but if you are the type of person who finds it impossible to eat just one cookie, you are better off staying away.

Processed Foods

Mental Help Net has a web site that exists to promote mental health and wellness education and advocacy. It has published an article[8] that discusses the impact of processed foods on the body. Here are some valuable excerpts from this article.

Your body needs both calories and nutrients to function properly. Unfortunately, not all foods provide quality nutrients. So-called "junk foods" (e.g., candy bars, sodas, fast-food hamburgers, etc.) are high in calories and in refined sugars and/or saturated fats, but do not provide worthwhile nutrients. While junk foods can be sources of quick energy, they are bad for overall health. A steady diet of junk food can actually contribute to malnutrition and disease.

Over the last century, food producers have taken to refining foods so that they will last longer on supermarket shelves. The process of refining food, however, often damages its nutritional value.

SixWise.com is a web site whose mission is to help you and your loved ones be safe, live longer, and prosper in all aspects of life by providing you with key insights, top recommendations, and practical solutions culled from the world's leading experts. The site's free newsletter[9] contains a great article titled "All the Health Risks of Processed Foods—In Just a Few Quick, Convenient Bites." Here are some excerpts from this very important article:

> Every day, 7 percent of the U.S. population visits a McDonald's, and between 20 and 25 percent of Americans eat fast food of some kind daily, says Steven Gortmaker, professor of society, human development, and health at the Harvard School of Public Health.

> But that's just the tip of the iceberg. Americans get processed food not only from fast-food restaurants but also from their neighborhood grocery stores. As it stands, about 90 percent of the money that Americans spend on food is used to buy processed foods.

> Think about it—if it comes in a box, can, bag, or carton, it's processed. The fact that these foods are so readily available and, often, of such poor quality, have led some, like associate professor of pediatrics at Harvard David Ludwig, to say that they're actually discouraging healthy eating and leading to a "toxic environment."

> "There's the incessant advertising and marketing of the poorest quality foods imaginable. To address this epidemic, you'd want to make healthful foods widely available, inexpensive, and convenient, and unhealthful foods relatively less so. Instead, we've done the opposite," says Ludwig.

> Processed foods have indeed been implicated in a host of chronic diseases and health conditions that are currently plaguing the nation. What follows is just a taste of the risks processed foods may present to your health.

> ### Obesity

> The World Health Organization (WHO) says processed foods are to blame for the sharp rise in obesity (and chronic disease) seen around the world. In

one study by Ludwig and colleagues, children who ate processed fast foods in a restaurant ate 126 more calories than on days they did not. Over the course of a year, this could translate into 13 pounds of weight gain just from fast food.

"The food industry would love to explain obesity as a problem of personal responsibility, since it takes the onus off them for marketing fast food, soft drinks, and other high-calorie, low-quality products," Ludwig says.

However, "When you have calories that are incredibly cheap, in a culture where "bigger is better," that's a dangerous combination," says Walter Willett, M.D., D.P.H., professor of epidemiology and nutrition at the Harvard School of Public Health.

Diabetes

"In the last 50 years, the extent of processing has increased so much that prepared breakfast cereals—even without added sugar—act exactly like sugar itself …

"As far as our hormones and metabolism are concerned, there's no difference between a bowl of unsweetened corn flakes and a bowl of table sugar. Starch is 100 percent glucose [table sugar is half glucose, half fructose] and our bodies can digest it into sugar instantly," says Ludwig.

"We are not adapted to handle fast-acting carbohydrates. Glucose is the gold standard of energy metabolism. The brain is exquisitely dependent on having a continuous supply of glucose: too low a glucose level poses an immediate threat to survival. [But] too high a level causes damage to tissues, as with diabetes," he continued.

Heart Disease

Many processed foods contain trans-fatty acids (TFA), a dangerous type of fat. According to the American Heart Association, "TFAs tend to raise LDL ("bad") cholesterol and lower HDL ("good") cholesterol. These changes may increase the risk of heart disease."

Further, most processed foods are extremely high in salt, another blow to the heart. A half-cup of Campbell's chicken noodle soup, for instance, has 37 percent of the daily-recommended amount of sodium.

"Probably the single fastest way to reduce the number of strokes in this country is to halve the amount of salt that's added to processed food," says Tim Lang, professor of food policy at the City University, London.

Cancer

A seven-year study of close to 200,000 people by the University of Hawaii found that people who ate the most processed meats (hot dogs, sausage) had a 67-percent-higher risk of pancreatic cancer than those who ate little or no meat products.

A Canadian study of over 400 men aged fifty to eighty found similar results. Men whose eating habits fell into the "processed" pattern (processed meats, red meat, organ meats, refined grains, vegetable oils, and soft drinks) had a significantly higher risk of prostate cancer than men in the other groups. Men who ate the most processed foods had a 2.5-fold increased prostate cancer risk.

Yet another study published in the journal *Cancer Epidemiology, Mile Markers, and Prevention* found that refined carbohydrates like white flour, sugar and high-fructose corn syrup are also linked to cancer. The study of more than 1,800 women in Mexico found that those who got 57 percent or more of their total energy intake from refined carbohydrates had a 220 percent higher risk of breast cancer than women who ate more balanced diets.

Processed meats like hot dogs, lunch meats, bacon, and sausages have been linked to various forms of cancer.

Acrylamide, a carcinogenic substance that forms when foods are heated at high temperatures, such as during baking or frying, is also a concern. Processed foods like french fries and potato chips have shown elevated levels of the substance, according to the Center for Science in the Public Interest (CSPI).

"I estimate that acrylamide causes several thousand cancers per year in Americans," said Clark University research professor Dale Hattis.

Is the convenience of food that is already packaged really worth the sacrifice of your health in exchange?

The George Mateljan Foundation, a nonprofit organization with no commercial interests, has an article on its web site entitled "What Are the Problems with Processed Foods?"[10] The foundation was established to help individuals discover, develop, and share scientifically proven information about the benefits of healthy eating. It believes that true good health is more than just the absence of disease; it is a state in which you enjoy all the energy, vitality, and benefits that life has to offer. Here are some important parts of the article:

Some of the many additives included in processed foods are thought to have the ability to compromise the body's structure and function. Therefore, avoiding foods that contain chemical additives may greatly contribute to your health and vitality.

Artificial Sweeteners

One of the most commonly used sweeteners is the controversial compound aspartame. Aspartame gains its controversy because animal studies have shown that it can lead to accumulation of formaldehyde after consumption, and one of the breakdown products of aspartame in the intestine is the toxic compound methanol. However, low levels of aspartame have not shown direct symptoms in humans, so it is presumed safe in food products. There is a problem with this assumption, though, because so many processed products contain aspartame, and therefore people who consume mainly processed foods may be taking in relatively high levels of aspartame.

Coloring Agents

Most processed foods are colored with synthetic or additional coloring agents. Based on the idea that we "eat with our eyes," many food manufactures choose to enhance a color, even if the initial food is not as colorful. Besides the issues of ingesting compounds that are not natural, colorings are often used to improve the color of foods that have lost color during storage or from heat. In sensitive persons, consumption of artificial colorings has been linked to ADHD (attention-deficit-hyperactivity disorder), asthma, and inflammatory skin conditions such as urticaria and atopic dermatitis.

Preservatives

A major concern with processed foods is the use of preservatives. The most commonly used preservatives are butylated hydroxytoluene (BHT) and sulfites.

Butylated Hydroxytoluene (BHT)

BHT is controversial. In 1978, a government-sponsored review of safety data indicated that no direct toxicity was observed at the permitted levels in a food. However, this report also determined that more studies were needed to assess safety. Since then, BHT has been shown to induce tumors in the stomach and liver in animals when used at high levels. Again, although it was allowed in foods at a low level per each food, it is one of the most common preservatives and is present in many processed foods. The amount consumed in a person's entire diet may be higher than the permitted level per food and remains a concern for many scientists.

Sulfites

Sulfites are also a common preservative. Sulfites are prohibited for use in foods that provide the nutrient vitamin B1 because it can destroy this vitamin. Furthermore, some people are sensitive to sulfites and respond with adverse reactions. Due to reports of adverse reactions, the FDA banned the use of sulfites on fruits and vegetables in 1986 and is still reviewing whether it should be banned from other uses.

Pesticides

The Environmental Protection Agency considers a number of herbicides and fungicides to be potentially carcinogenic and therefore able to cause genetic damage leading to the development of cancer. Most pesticides are known to cause some risk to humans. Both the Natural Resources Defense Council and the Environmental Working Group have found that millions of Americans are exposed to levels of pesticides in their food that exceed limits considered to be safe.

Trans-Fats

Trans-fatty acids are an example of what can happen to essential nutrients when a food is processed. Also called hydrogenated fats, these fatty acids are found in margarine, vegetable shortenings, crackers, cookies, snack foods and numerous other processed foods. Trans-fats are produced by a chemical process in which hydrogen is added to an unsaturated fatty acid. The food industry uses this process because it converts a liquid fat to a soft solid form, like margarine, and also because it increases the shelf-life of fats.

In this process, however, the fatty acid molecule shifts structures to one that is not found in the body; that is, the fats in the body occur in what is called a "cis" 3-dimensional structure, and trans-fatty acids occur in the opposite of that—a "trans" structure. Chemically, they are different. Your body notices this difference. Although you may think that the fat you are eating will support your body's functioning, it instead is a different structure than the one that your body needs. Your body has a different response to trans-fats.

Trans-fats have been shown to increase LDL cholesterol (the one associated with increased risk of heart disease) and decrease HDL cholesterol, the "protective" cholesterol. So clear is the promotion of high LDL cholesterol levels by trans-fats and the resultant association with increased risk for heart disease, that the FDA has been prompted to require these trans-fats be labeled separately on foods, so that consumers can see when they are present. Trans-fats have also been linked to certain cancers, including breast cancer, and labeling them allows you to see how often they are used in processed foods, thereby allowing you to avoid these foods.

Practical Tip

All of these compounds, just to make food look and taste as close to natural as possible. Why not buy a natural, whole food and not all these synthetics? Real food has real benefits …

Fad Diets

When you eat what you want when you want it, sooner or later there is a consequence to your actions. One day you wake up and notice that your clothes don't fit as well as they used to anymore. Your pants won't close. Your jacket is snug. "Maybe the dry cleaner shrunk my clothes," you say to yourself. But inside, you know what has happened. You've been eating too much. You are sluggish. Your energy is down. It's time to do something about it.

In the instant-gratification society that we live in, you will want to lose the weight as quickly as possible. Even though the weight was gained slowly, and therefore must come off slowly, you won't want to wait. You will reach for solutions that you believe will show results immediately. You'll turn on the TV and see a commercial for a program that will claim to help you drop thirty pounds in a month. Or you will have a conversation with a co-worker who lost a lot of weight fast, and you will want to go on that program too.

Welcome to the world of fad dieting that will give you hope. Do some fad diets work? Yes. If you stop eating, you will lose weight. But what happens when you get hungry? What happens when willpower is not enough? What happens when your energy level is low because you are not eating enough? In these cases, you will likely binge and gain more than you lost. Hopelessness will return, and the cycle and quest to lose weight quickly will continue—no matter what fad dieting is doing to your body and mental heath.

The American Academy of Family Physicians had an article titled "Fad Diets: What You Need to Know"[11] on familydoctor.org. Here are some of their informative points about fad dieting.

What Is a Fad Diet?

A fad diet is a weight loss plan or aid that promises dramatic results. These diets don't offer long-term success, and they are usually not very healthy. Some of them can actually be dangerous to your health.

If Fad Diets Don't Work, Why Are They So Popular?

People are often willing to try anything that promises to help them lose weight because they want to look or feel better, or because they are worried about getting weight-related diseases. Companies that promote fad diets take advantage of this fact. They appeal to people by promising weight loss that's very quick and easy. Many people prefer to try the quick fix of a fad diet instead of making the effort to lose weight through long-term changes in their eating and exercise habits.

Fad diets also become popular because many of them do work for a short time. In many cases, this is because when you stop eating certain types of food or eat "special" combinations of foods, you are getting fewer calories than you normally would. You are also paying more attention to what you are eating. However, it's likely that much of the weight you lose is from water and lean muscle, not body fat. Also, most people are not able to keep up with the demands of a diet that strictly limits their food choices or requires them to eat the same foods over and over again. People who use fad diets usually end up gaining back any weight that they lost.

You can't have high energy if you are hungry.

Stress

Workplace stress causes about one million U.S. employees to miss work each day.[12]

Health.com, a health and wellness magazine, gives women useful and up-to-date information and inspiration on how to live healthier and happier lives. Recently they featured an article[13] about job stress. Here are some important points from that article.

> One-fourth of employees view their jobs as the number one stressor in their lives. *Northwestern National Life*

> Three-fourths of employees believe the worker has more on-the-job stress than a generation ago. *Princeton Survey Research Associates*

> Problems at work are more strongly associated with health complaints than are any other life stressor-more so than even financial problems or family problems. *St. Paul Fire and Marine Insurance Company*

What Is Job Stress?

Job stress can be defined as the harmful physical and emotional responses that occur when the requirements of the job do not match the capabilities, resources, or needs of the worker. Job stress can lead to poor health and even injury.

The concept of job stress is often confused with challenge, but these concepts are not the same. Challenge energizes us psychologically and physically, and it motivates us to learn new skills and master our jobs. When a challenge is met, we feel relaxed and satisfied. Challenge is an important ingredient for healthy and productive work.

What Are The Causes Of Job Stress?

Nearly everyone agrees that job stress results from the interaction between the worker and the conditions of work. Views differ, however, on the importance of worker characteristics versus working conditions as the primary cause of job stress. These differing viewpoints are important because they suggest different ways to prevent stress at work.

According to one school of thought, differences in individual characteristics such as personality and coping style are most important in predicting whether certain job conditions will result in stress—in other words, what is stressful for one person may not be a problem for someone else. This viewpoint leads to prevention strategies that focus on workers and ways to help them cope with demanding job conditions.

Although the importance of individual differences cannot be ignored, scientific evidence suggests that certain working conditions are stressful to most people. Excessive workload demands and conflicting expectations are good examples. Such evidence argues for a greater emphasis on working conditions as the key source of job stress, and for job redesign as a primary prevention strategy.

In 1960, a Michigan court upheld a compensation claim by an automotive assembly-line worker who had difficulty keeping up with the pressures of the production line. To avoid falling behind, he tried to work on several assemblies at the same time and often got parts mixed up. As a result, he was subjected to repeated criticism from the foreman. Eventually he suffered a psychological breakdown.—1995 Workers Compensation Yearbook

Job Conditions That May Lead to Stress

- The Design of Tasks. Heavy workload; infrequent rest breaks; long work hours; shift work; hectic and routine tasks that have little inherent meaning, do not utilize workers' skills, and provide little sense of control.

- Management Style. Lack of participation by workers in decision-making; poor communication in the organization; lack of family-friendly policies.

- Interpersonal Relationships. Poor social environment and lack of support or help from co-workers and supervisors.

- Work Roles. Conflicting or uncertain job expectations; too much responsibility; too many "hats to wear."

- Career Concerns. Job insecurity and lack of opportunity for growth, advancement, or promotion; rapid changes for which workers are unprepared.

- Environmental Conditions. Unpleasant or dangerous physical conditions such as crowding, noise, air pollution, or ergonomic problems.

Early Warning Signs of Stress

- Headache

- Sleep Disturbances

- Difficulty in Concentrating

- Short Temper

- Upset Stomach

- Job Dissatisfaction

- Low Morale

Job Stress and Health

Stress sets off an alarm in the brain, which responds by preparing the body for defensive action. The nervous system is aroused and hormones are released to sharpen the senses, quicken the pulse, deepen respiration, and tense the muscles. This response (sometimes called the fight-or-flight response) is important because it helps us defend against threatening situations. The response is preprogrammed biologically. Everyone responds in much the same way, regardless of whether the stressful situation is at work or home.

Short-lived or infrequent episodes of stress pose little risk. But when stressful situations go unresolved, the body is kept in a constant state of activation, which increases the rate of wear and tear to biological systems. Ultimately, fatigue or damage results, and the ability of the body to repair and defend itself can become seriously compromised. As a result, the risk of injury or disease escalates.

Many studies have looked at the relationship between job stress and a variety of ailments. Mood and sleep disturbances, upset stomach and headache, and disturbed relationships with family and friends are examples of stress-related problems that are quick to develop and are commonly seen in these studies. These early signs of job stress are usually easy to recognize. But the effects of job stress on chronic diseases are more difficult to see because chronic diseases take a long time to develop and can be influenced by many factors other than stress. Nonetheless, evidence is rapidly accumulating to suggest that stress plays an important role in several types of chronic health problems—especially cardiovascular disease, musculoskeletal disorders, and psychological disorders.

Stress can hurt your career. If you are wound up, worried, and overworked, it will be hard for you to feel good about your career and have the energy to advance it. Once you have identified what is stressing you, you can create a plan to change it.

Disorganization

In an article written for the *Boston Business Journal*, Marilyn Paul[14], author of the book *It's Hard to Make a Difference When You Can't Find Your Keys*, discusses ways in which businesses are disorganized.

What does a disorganized workplace look and feel like? Here's what a few people in such organizations had to say:

"We are overwhelmed and exhausted. We push hard to get through one project, and then there's another one that we have to do," says a manager of a biotech organization.

"We race to get products out the door, but often we find major errors because we have been pushing so hard and everyone is tired. Then there is the major push to rectify the error, plus the yelling and blaming and trying to figure out who did the bad deed," says the operations manager of a manufacturing plant.

"We e-mail everyone to keep them informed, then nobody has time to read their e-mails. A typical day leaves me with 200 e-mail messages in my inbox" says a marketing director of a major pharmaceutical company.

"I can't trust anyone here to do what they say they are going to do. I like them, and we are all friendly, but I can't count on anyone. If you want to get anything done around here, you have to do it yourself," says a foundation director.

"This place is a mess. People leave dirty coffee cups in the kitchen, there are dead plants in the window, and someone left a bunch of boxes in the closet. We can't agree on how to keep this place looking nice," says the receptionist at a startup.

"I don't have one moment during the day to stop and reflect on what we are doing or why we are doing it," says a management consultant.

Where are you focusing your energies? On other people's mistakes, or on what you can do to be more productive? What does your desk look like? Your in-box? Can you find things easily? How many unfinished projects can you complete? Disorganization can throw you off balance and make you feel out of control.

Lack Of Physical Activity

Many jobs today require people to sit all day. This means that slumping over your desk is what your body has grown used to. The truth is your body will ache more if it's in the same position all day. Movement will make you feel better and increase your energy level.

The U.S. Department of Health and Human Services issued a report[15] showing that seven in ten American adults are not regularly active, including four in ten who are not active at all.

An article on the SeniorJournal.com web site entitled "Lack of Physical Activity More Life Threatening than Obesity"[16] discusses how not exercising can increase your mortality risk. An important point the article makes is that being inactive is more life-threatening than being overweight or obese.

There can always be a reason not to move your body if you let there be one. You are busy. You are tired. There is no time to exercise. Are your reasons keeping you from being in the best shape you can be? If so, remember that it's not fun walking around feeling tired and achy. If you want more energy, you need to get moving.

Lack Of Sleep

"It's unfortunate that in our 24-7 society, sleep is viewed as expendable and something you can catch up on anytime. The trouble is many of us don't catch up on lost sleep."

—Richard L. Gelula, executive director of the National Sleep Foundation.[17]

Do you think that you are the only one who struggles to make it through the day? Think again.

The independent and nonprofit National Sleep Foundation,[18] located in Washington DC, published a survey of 1,154 adults that reported the following:

- More than half of workers surveyed—51 percent—said that being tired on the job interferes with the amount of work they get done and affects their performance in several ways. Concentrating was harder for 68 percent of respondents; handling stress was more difficult for 65 percent; problem-solving and decision-making was harder for 58 percent; and listening to co-workers was more of a chore for 57 percent.

- More than a quarter of those questioned—27 percent—said that they were tired at work two or more days per week. Women admitted to tiredness more often than men——31 percent vs. 22 percent. Young people aged eighteen to twenty-nine complained most of work-related tiredness, with 40 percent saying that it was a problem at least twice a week.

- Almost one in five workers—19 percent—said that she or he occasionally or frequently made mistakes at work because of tiredness. Well above the average in this category were sales workers at 35 percent, retail workers at 33 percent, and financial, insurance, and real-estate professionals at 29 percent.

- Of those surveyed, nearly one in seven—14 percent—said that he or she was occasionally or frequently late to work because of tiredness. For young workers in the eighteen-to-twenty-nine age range, the figure was 22 percent.

Not sleeping well at night will make you more tired during the day, and your work and energy level will suffer. You can't feel your best if you are sleepy.

Overwork

How many items do you have on your to-do list? Does it empower you to look at your list, or are you drained before you even try to accomplish the first task? Of course, a to-do list can help you get organized and focused. But ask yourself: Are you controlling your to-do list, or is your to-do list controlling you?

If you are controlled by your to-do list—if it feels as though your sanity depends on the number of items you check off—then it may no longer be a useful tool. Instead, it may be a source of stress and frustration and may be standing in the way of achieving what you want in your career.

Could your to-do list be so long because you are forcing yourself to do too much work? Are you working extra-long hours, working in your free time, taking work home with you, working on your vacation, and checking your e-mail right before you go to bed and first thing when you rise? Has your job become your life?

Randall S. Hansen, PhD, webmaster at Quintessential Careers, as well as publisher of its electronic newsletter, *QuintZine*, has written an article titled "Are You—or Someone You Know—a Workaholic?"[19] Here's what the article says about the amount of time we spend working.

> Americans are working more hours per week than in years past, and with all the downsizings and consolidations and lack of replacement hiring, more and more workers are putting in extra hours to complete the work previously completed by others. Some studies show that as much as many as 40 percent of workers don't even bother to take vacations, partly because of fears they may not have a job to come back to if they do.
>
> We live and work in a connected environment—e-mails, instant messaging, fax machines, cell phones, and digital assistants—making it hard for workers to truly get time away from their work.
>
> Whether it is how more and more of us mistakenly define success in terms of financial and materialistic measures or the fact that many Americans simply must work multiple jobs simply to earn a living wage and keep their families out of poverty, we are working more and more for the financial outcomes.

It would be much easier to work less if working hard weren't so well rewarded. Promotions and higher pay go to those who spend more time at their desks.

Furthermore, when you are working on a big project, there is often a pleasurable rush; and close friendships can be formed when you are a part of a team. There is also a feeling of pride when you are good at what you do.

Nevertheless, working *too* much can negate all of these benefits. Working too much can turn you into a workaholic. How do you know if you are a workaholic? A workaholic is someone with a compulsive and unrelenting need to work. Is this you? Whether you are working too much because you want to, or because you feel that you have no choice, working all the time will drain your energy.

According to a *Fast Company* magazine article titled "My Name Is Tony, and I'm A Workaholic,"[20] writer Tony Schwartz, author of *What Really Matters: Searching for Wisdom in America* says:

> Working 24–7 takes a toll. A survey by the American Academy of Matrimonial Lawyers cited preoccupation with work as one of the top four causes of divorce. Workaholics themselves evidence more destructive behavior: more alcohol abuse, more extramarital affairs, and more stress-related illnesses.

But companies continue to demand more work produced at a faster rate. And why shouldn't they? It benefits them enormously.

In an article titled "Business Benefits from Workaholic Managers"[21] posted to the Personnel Today web site, the benefits of a constantly working workforce were discussed:

> A Chartered Management Institute (CMI) survey of more than 6,000 managers found that more than half (54 percent) contact their organization by choice during holidays due to work overload. More than two-thirds (68 percent) also respond to requests from their employer while on leave.

> This is despite the fact that employers encourage staff to have time off, with 66 percent of respondents reporting more than five weeks holiday entitlement, up from 56 percent in 2003.

> Even when they finally go on holiday, managers find it difficult to relax. Almost half (48 percent) regularly check their work e-mail and 43 percent monitor voicemail. In an effort to keep in touch with colleagues, 57 percent

take away their work mobile phones, 20 percent take their laptops, and 14 percent regularly visit internet cafes.

If you find that your life is out of balance, look at the amount of time you spend in the office. You can't continue at a fast pace forever. Sooner or later, your energy level will decrease, and interests outside of the office will play an important role to raise it.

Unhealed Emotions

The longer you work, the greater the chance of painful things happening to you in your career. Maybe you get fired for no reason. Perhaps you are passed over for a promotion you deserved. Maybe you become unemployed or the victim of mass layoffs. Maybe you have a terrible boss. Everyone has a story to tell, and each story hurts.

Nursing unhealed emotions in the workplace will sap your energy. You may decide not to take your career to the next level because of something that happened to you in the past. You may think that unfortunate events in the past will carry over into the future. This kind of thinking has no basis in fact. The past does not necessarily predict the future; but if you dwell too much on the past, you will raise the chances of recreating it. You must let go of hurtful episodes from the past before you can design a career for your present and future—one that brings you enjoyment and satisfaction.

The Executive Connection (TEC) is an international organization that provides continuous learning, mentoring, and development for chief executives, managing directors, and business owners in a peer group setting. It has an article on its web site written by Barton Goldsmith, PhD, titled "There's No Crying in Baseball: The Truth about Emotions in Business."[22] Here are some excerpts from that article:

> One of the ways negative emotions present themselves in the workplace is when team members withdraw and are unavailable to themselves and their co-workers. This is a reaction to hurt feelings incurred from in and out of the workplace. To put it in Psych 101 terms: People act out their pain.
>
> When people get their feelings hurt, they can become unconscious saboteurs. This can manifest in a number of ways including not contributing at

meetings, missing deadlines, and even offending clients. Ninety-nine percent of the time, this is an unconscious behavior. People are not aware they are doing it since the unconscious mind controls 90 percent of their actions. If unhealed emotions are not addressed, there will be significant losses in terms of personnel, a dwindling customer base, financial success, and market positioning.

These losses in addition to the loss of your health and fulfillment may occur. Are unhealed emotions hurting you?

Being A Lone Ranger

One of the biggest mistakes I see as a career coach is people wanting to handle their career challenges alone. Below is an excerpt from an article I wrote titled "Stop Tackling Your Career Alone"[23] that outlines why we feel that we need to handle career problems by ourselves. The article was published on 6figurejobs.com, a leading online executive career portal.

> Reaching out is so hard that many people would prefer to search for what they need in their careers on their own, rather than ask for help. They go for months or years without a solution, until they cannot take it anymore. Then they have to ask for help out of desperation.
>
> Life is not about reaching our goals alone. When we try to overcome a challenge by ourselves, we have to battle our inner demons (our worries, fears, anxieties, etc.) single-handedly, which in most cases is unsuccessful. Other people (fortunately) do not see us as we see ourselves. In times of doubt, we need them to remind us of our greatness.
>
> Life is about give and take. Right now you need something. It's OK to ask for assistance. The person who helps you today might be the person who asks for your help tomorrow. Seasons change, and so do the cycles in our careers. Sometimes we are soaring, and at other times we are confused and disappointed. Know that this cycle will end one day, and success is right around the corner.
>
> If you are worried that someone in your life might not want to help you, let him or her tell you that. Don't assume they will think less of you for opening up and sharing an aspect of your career that is not going well at the moment. The only one who is embarrassed is you. The people who truly care about you will be honored that you asked for their opinion and guidance.

You are not alone, and this is one of the many reasons why I wrote this book. There are more people experiencing energy and work troubles than you think.

Job Dissatisfaction

Are you unhappy at work?

Here are some important facts to remember:

- When you are doing what you love to do, you are happy, excited, and full of energy.
- If you love your job, the other areas in your life will improve dramatically.

It's difficult to feel unhappy at work. After a while, you start to believe that you are trapped and cannot do anything about your situation. Negative thoughts take root and grow stronger over time. They can do real damage. They can affect every area of your life, including your relationships, motivation, physical health, and mental well-being. If being unhappy at work does so much damage, then why do many people stay in jobs that make them unhappy for so long? Mostly, it's because they are afraid.

If you are unhappy in your job, what thoughts come to mind when you think about getting another one? Do you worry that the grass may not be greener on the other side? Do you wonder whether you will be able to pay your bills? Do you worry that you may make a mistake and end up in a similar situation as the one you are in now?

You may be unhappy and know it's time to change your job (or career), yet you may believe that the known is preferable to the unknown. You may continue along the same path and hope that the road will improve on its own. This is a mistake. Not only will you continue to suffer emotionally, but your spirits and self-esteem will diminish while you are waiting for the situation to change.

Is being happy in a job really that important? Yes.

In an article that I wrote that was published on columbuswired.net—Central Ohio's Premier Online Magazine—I discussed the signs that may suggest that you are in the wrong job/career.[24] Here is the article:

Are you happy when you come to work in the morning, or happy when it is time to go home? Do you look forward to Friday and then get knots in your stomach on Sunday evenings? If this is the case, there is probably nothing wrong with you physically. You may be in the wrong job.

Most people view their lives as being separate parts: work life/social life/home life. Your life has many components, but when you are in the wrong job, the rest of your life is out of balance.

So, how do you know if you are in the wrong job? Ask yourself the following:

1. Do I have a hard time falling asleep at night?

Are you so wound up at the end of the day that you cannot seem to calm down at night? If you are playing the same thoughts in your head over and over again, you are probably trying to get closure for the day. You could also be trying to make sense of what is happening around you. If you were in the right job, you would fall asleep more easily.

2. Do I have trouble making it to work on time?

Most of the time, being late does not happen by accident. Yes, outside circumstances could be the reason you are not getting to work on time, but your lateness is probably a result of you not wanting to be there. If you were in the right job, you would make it to work on time.

3. Do I feel run-down?

Have you put on weight recently? Have you stopped exercising? Do you get frequent headaches, stomachaches, or colds? These are tell-tale signs that your job is taking away from your quality of life. If you were in the right job, you would not be punishing your body like you are.

4. Do I wish I were somewhere else?

If you wish you were somewhere else, then it may be time to make a plan to get yourself there. There does not have to be anything wrong with you for wanting something different. If your inner voice is screaming for more, it may be time to listen. If you were in the right job, you might think about doing something else, but not all the time.

5. Do I believe that there is nothing I can do about my situation?

When you are in the wrong job, you lose the ability to see a way out. You become consumed with your unhappiness and forget that something better is around the corner. If you were in the right job, your thinking would be clearer.

Nothing will drain your energy more at work than job dissatisfaction. Know that no matter where you are in your career, you can change it for the better.

THE ANSWER

The answer is not to make a quick radical change. It's altering one thing at a time—making it easier to create lasting change that will stick. Making gradual changes will make it easier for you to become aware of them as they happen, giving you a more active role in solving your energy problem.

Let's begin with what you are eating. Are you eating real or processed food? Are you reading labels? Do you understand what you are putting into your body? Food is your fuel, and you want your body and mind to run on the best fuel possible. Having that in mind, start a food journal. (You can use the example provided.) Use it to become aware of what you are eating. Once you know what substances are entering your body, you will more easily be able to make different, better choices. You can't change what you are eating until you know what to change.

Food Journal Example

Date	Meal #1	Snack #1	Meal #2	Snack #2	Meal #3	Snack #3	Water Intake (ounces)	Exercise

As you keep track of your eating habits, on the same chart, keep track of how active you are. Are you moving your body as much as you'd like? Having the answer written down in front of you is empowering. Once you see more clearly what you need to do, it will be much easier to actually do it.

How are you spending your time? Keep a record of that, too. (You can use the example provided.) You may be surprised to discover that there is more time available to you than you thought. Once you know what you are doing with your time, it will be easier to make different choices about how to spend it.

Time Tracking Journal Example

Date _____

Time of Task   **Tasks** _____

_____

_____

_____

_____

_____

_____

_____

_____

_____

_____

_____

_____

_____

It's essential that you make time for *you*. If you were to spend fifteen minutes every day doing something for yourself, even that short amount of time would make you feel better and more relaxed.

This section of the book was loaded with information to help you become aware of what you may be doing to your mind and body at your job and because of it. Yes, work is important. But if you get sick (or are sick) because you are not taking good care of yourself, you may come to regret putting so much emphasis on your job, at the expense of your health.

There was also a lot of information in this section about the sorts of things you should *not* do. At times, reading this type of information can be overpowering, to the point at which you begin to shut it out. By doing this, you may prevent yourself from being overwhelmed; but you may also be keeping out information that is important for you to know. This is why it is essential to have all the facts, even if some of them may be unpleasant. Often, you can't change what's happening around you, but with the correct information, you can still change your own actions for the better. I suspect that if you really understood the unhealthy things you were regularly putting into and doing to your body and the consequences that might result, it would amaze, if not frighten you. You would probably stop immediately. I hope that you will be able to use this book to help you do just that.

Step 2:
Decide To Change

"I Matter"

Earlier in her career, Michelle had been a top nurse in a top hospital. She was a rising star—happy, energetic, and successful. Michelle had a good life, a loving husband, and was in great shape. She had it all. Then she and her husband decided to start a family. Sadly, she had three miscarriages before she got pregnant a fourth time. Michelle's fourth pregnancy involved many complications, and she was put on bed rest. Her baby was born with a breathing disorder, which led to brain damage. The baby died a month and a half later.

That's when Michelle seemed to become one of the living dead. Going through the motions, yet not really living. Despite what had happened, Michelle and her husband kept trying to have kids. Eventually, Michelle had two difficult pregnancies that resulted in two healthy babies. She was happy to be a mom, but something felt wrong inside. At this point, she started overeating and the scale began to rise. Of course, a certain amount of weight gain came with the pregnancies, but her lifestyle after her children were born prevented the weight from coming off. Michelle knew she was getting heavier, but she didn't care. She had a high-stress job and was going back to school to get her master's degree, so it was easier for her to eat what was available, rather than seeking out healthier alternatives. Michelle ate at her desk, ingesting her food quickly. She ate a lot of candies and cookies. She ate too much fast food. Sometimes, she would choose healthy snacks, but eat too much of them, enabling the weight gain to continue.

One day, Michelle was watching a talk show on television. The host asked a woman who was having a hard time in her life, "What changed for you? What was the moment when your life changed and you turned down the wrong path?" This question hit Michelle hard. She realized that for her, this moment was the death of her baby many years earlier. This terrible event had changed her from a happy person into an unhappy one. After realizing this, Michelle made the decision to change, to tell herself that she mattered, and that her obesity was due to her failure to take care of herself.

Michelle joined a gym and exercised regularly. She started eating balanced meals. In the evenings, Michelle would decide what she would eat at work the next day. She would prepare raw vegetable snacks ahead of time, so that they would be ready for her to take to work in the morning. She stopped taking phone calls while eating lunch, so that she could enjoy her food undisturbed. If there was a celebration at work, she would only have a small piece of cake. Michelle accepted that work often entails stress and conflict, and that the demands it tries to place on you may exceed what you can reasonably be expected to accomplish. She learned to disregard the things she could not fix—such as other people's difficult personalities—and focused on fixing what she could, like her own attitude. Michelle eventually left her job and started a business of her own. Today, she takes care of herself first and feels much better, both physically and mentally, than when she was younger.

Michelle lost 112 pounds over a two-year period. Her weight loss and pathway to better health began when she decided that she mattered and wanted to be healthy again.

CHOOSE ENERGY

Work can be frustrating and stressful. Sometimes, if your work goes unacknowledged, you can feel like a number instead of a person. At other times, you may feel that your work is not making a difference. At meetings, you may present ideas that no one seems to listen to. You may write reports that never get read. You want to improve the way things are done in your workplace, but may feel like you are the only one who cares.

One of the biggest problems associated with work frustration is that it often leads people to take these frustrations out on themselves. Rather than finding a constructive way to release negative feelings and emotions, they often prefer to escape and not think about them. This technique may provide temporary relief; but it can never deal with the challenges at work that cause the frustration in the first place. In many cases, ignoring problems only makes them worse.

No matter how tough your job is, you'll need a healthy mind and body to confront it. If you are eating poorly, not exercising, or internalizing stress, you won't feel well. And if you don't feel well, you can't treat your career with the attention and respect it deserves. Without energy, you cannot make your career as fulfilling as it could be.

Many people tell me that it's not possible to love one's job. "Work is work," they say. "You don't have to love what you do. Work is done to pay the bills. Weekends and evenings are the only times you can truly enjoy life." To put it bluntly, this is obviously wrong. It *is* possible to love what you do for a living. I've helped thousands of people learn how to love their careers, so I know it can be done. But if you have low energy, this learning process can be much more difficult. With increased energy, you will give yourself the best chance of having a career you love. With energy, it can feel as though anything is possible.

> Choosing energy means discarding what doesn't work, so that you can make room for what does.

The following are changes you can make to allow high energy and passion to become driving forces in your career.

LET GO OF RESISTANCE

There are times in your career when what you want is not aligned with what you are getting. Maybe you want a harmonious work environment, but you have co-workers who drive you crazy. Maybe you want a new position, but are being consistently passed over for promotion. Maybe you want a raise or greater recognition for your efforts, but find other people taking credit for your work.

Instead of taking action to get more energy to help you change your circumstances, you find yourself waiting for the situation to improve on its own. And while you are waiting, you keep hurting yourself by eating foods that you know are not good for you, by sitting at your desk all day without taking a break, and by keeping stress bottled up inside. When you resist, harmful habits persist. You may not have the motivation to do something different, but this deficit must be overcome. You cannot build up your energy without some type of change. You have to stop resisting what you know you need to do. By doing so, you will be taking the first step toward getting healthy again.

Decide to stop resisting solutions you have been seeing as "impossible," and you may be surprised to discover how possible they've been all along.

LET GO OF ANGER

Anger is a normal emotion. Some things have happened (and will happen) to you in your career that you will not like. This is true for everyone. Often, it's not what actually happens, but how you react to it that is detrimental to your state of mind. How you choose to channel your anger can affect your well-being.

I have clients who can remember something hurtful that a co-worker said to them ten years ago. Or who still brood over a job they wanted long ago that was given to someone who did not deserve it. Some can pinpoint a moment in the distant past that was the reason why their careers took a turn for the worse. I know that these moments hurt. But whatever may have happened, realize that it was probably not purposely done to hurt you. At times, it can seem that there are people who are out to "get" you; but the truth is that most people act foolishly because they don't know any better, or because fear and stress have driven them to use hurtful tactics.

When you cling to a painful emotion such as anger, you cannot feel energized. When you free yourself of angry thoughts, by forgiving yourself and others, you will free up a lot of mental space which can be filled with newfound energy.

Decide to let your anger go, so you can improve your chances of feeling great.

LET GO OF BLAME

Who do you blame when something goes wrong at work? Your incompetent co-workers or boss? The outrageous deadline for the project you are working on? The company's culture or politics?

Let me suggest that no one is to blame. Rather, someone is responsible. Is it possible that the responsible person is you? What I mean to say is that the person who controls how you feel about what's happening is you.

We are a society of blamers. We all do it. Even though we criticize others for not taking responsibility, when it's our turn to be responsible, we tend to look outward to assign blame if something goes wrong. Blame feels good, because we don't like to admit being wrong. The downside to blame is that it allows you to stay stuck and stagnant when you could actively be trying to improve the situation. In the end, relying on blame will make you feel worse. When you feel that you have been wronged, you have a decision to make: either insist on being right (and stuck); or keep moving, and find away around those who would hinder you.

Blame will drag down your energy level. If something at work is not going well, it is preferable to accept what is happening and try to learn from it. This way, you can make progress.

Decide against the easy solution of assigning blame. When you choose not to blame, a sense of calm can emerge, which will in turn help you to feel great, motivated, and empowered.

CHANGE YOUR BELIEFS

Your beliefs are powerful. They set the tone and direction for your career. If you say that you want one thing, but actually believe another, the resulting conflict will hold you back. Belief is critical to victory. If you do not believe that you can have a high level of energy in your career, then you are unlikely to achieve it.

Your beliefs about your present situation help to explain why you are where you are today. For example, if you believe that you cannot eat better during the day and that you are a slave to the foods around you, then you will not be energized. You will feel tired and have health problems. If you believe that there is no time to exercise, or that you are incapable of greater physical activity, then you will be out of shape. Because of this belief, you will feel older than you are. If you believe that you cannot do anything about stress, then you will feel agitated most of the time. If you retain such beliefs, you will not be able to advance in your life or in your career. Your view of your career will become negative, even though such feelings are the result not of your career, but of your beliefs.

Belief comes from within. Think back to times in your career when you believed you would be successful. Is there a difference in your beliefs then and now? You can believe in positive outcomes even if your plans for them haven't been fully realized yet.

Decide to let go of the beliefs that no longer serve you. Instead, focus on believing that you can transform yourself into a healthy, energetic person.

CHANGE YOUR ATTITUDE

Your career can be compared to a journey. As with any journey, there will be highs and lows along the way, in this case, spread out over many years. When good things are happening in your career, it will be easier to feel energized. But when more challenging things are occurring, it will naturally be more difficult to manage your energy efficiently.

Your attitude directly influences your reaction to stressful situations. Your attitude toward a given situation often influences your behavior more than the situation itself. Therefore, pay at least as much attention to your attitude as you do to the problems at hand. Try to replace a negative attitude with a will to succeed. If you can do this, you will no doubt see your energy-level soar.

Decide that your frustrations will not keep you from being in the best possible mental and physical health. You can't let frustration stand in the way of a bright future filled with lots of energy. One way to reduce a negative attitude is to write down a few positive affirmations and think about them every day. When you question your abilities, or doubt whether higher energy is possible, use this list to lift your spirits and return yourself to a more positive frame of mind.

MAKE BETTER CHOICES

Your career is filled with choices. Some of them will empower you, and others will hold you back. Setbacks in your career—one cause of low energy—usually arise not by accident, but as a result of the choices you've made.

For example:

- You choose to complete a project on your own. This choice holds you back because you are alienating others, rather than building a supportive network. Not only have you lost valuable allies, you have also needlessly caused yourself to work harder.

- You choose to send e-mails when you are angry. This choice holds you back because co-workers remember your rash decisions, thus straining your relationships with them.

- You choose to work excessively long hours. This choice holds you back because your hectic schedule drains your energy, clouds your perspective, and casts a shadow over your relationships. It creates an unbalanced life.

- You choose to coast through your career. This choice holds you back because your lack of passion will surely lead to lack of focus and direction.

All of these poor choices, and many others like them, will weigh you down.

Of course, no one intentionally makes bad choices. Every time you ate something that did not nourish your body, or skipped a workout, you probably made what you thought was the best choice at the time. You weighed your options and believed that you were doing the right thing. When you learn to question choices that are bad for you, you can also learn to make better choices in the future.

At the same time, it's important to make peace with your past choices. Closing the door on old, poor choices will make it easier to open another door to better ones. You cannot go back, but you can go forward. What choices are you making today? What choices are you continuing to make even though you know they are not good for you? Do you know in your heart that it's time to make healthy choices, but still hesitate?

Decide to make better choices. This is a vital step toward creating a healthy, energetic new you.

SHOULD YOU CHANGE YOUR JOB?

Does your job increase your energy or drain it from you?

Many people stay in their jobs longer than they want to, because they are unsure of what to do next. They tell themselves that the answer will come someday. Whenever that day comes, they will make their move. But in the meantime, they are stagnant and unhappy.

Your job will not get better until you make it better, or until you choose a new one. If you want to find a job you enjoy, one that empowers and energizes you, you will have to actively work at finding it. Yes, this may be challenging at times. But isn't staying in a job that is draining your energy and detracting from your quality of life even harder in the long run?

Decide to change your job if you are unhappy in the one you have now and you have given it your best shot.

SHOULD YOU CHANGE YOUR CAREER?

Are you in a career you love, or in a career you are tolerating?

What's the difference? If you're working strictly to earn a paycheck that will pay the bills, you are merely tolerating your career. But if your days are filled with passion and delight for the work you do, you have a dream career—one you are in love with.

Do you know in your heart that you want a career that gives you meaning, purpose, and satisfaction? If so, listen to your inner voice—it is trying to prompt you into action. When you get to a point in your career when you know it is not working for you anymore, it is important to make a change. Your energy depends on it.

Decide to change careers if your work drains you of energy or if you don't enjoy the work anymore.

Step 3:
Create Your High-Energy Vision

After you have decided to have more energy in your career, it's time to begin your journey toward obtaining it. All of life's journeys begin with the phrase, "I want." Think about your career and the times when you said "I want." Maybe you said "I want" to go to college—and then enrolled in school and completed your degree. Maybe you said "I want" to work for a large or a small company—and you are working there now. Maybe you said "I want" to lead teams—and that's one of your current responsibilities. "I want" is a very powerful phrase. Without it, it's hard to go very far.

You can't reach your destination until you know what it is.

Imagine going on a trip without selecting a destination beforehand. What would you pack? How would you get there? Where would you stay? Your trip probably would not end up being much fun.

It's the same with your career. Not being able to visualize your desired result leads to results not happening. Goals are reached when you decide what you want, and then take action to get it. Without an end in mind, you will wander aimlessly; and as long as you are aimless, you will be wasting time. You will feel lost. You will be like a stray leaf, going wherever the wind takes you. If your goal is high energy and feeling great at work every day, then it is important to create a picture in your mind of what this would be like.

All goals are reached in the mind first. You see yourself achieving that goal and can feel the happiness it will bring you once you are there. This picture is what will help you to persevere during times of doubt, or when results may not come as fast as you'd like. Your picture of success will give you purpose, power, and excitement. Your picture will give you a reason to get out of bed every day.

WHAT IS A HIGH-ENERGY VISION?

My definition of a vision is a visualization or a picture of where you see yourself in the future. Your picture can be one of where you want to be in a day, a week, a month, a year, or even farther into the future. The visualization of your goal is what compels you to move forward. A high-energy vision is a snapshot of what you want to look like and feel like in the future. This snapshot gives your journey a clear and reachable destination and provides focus.

You can create a high-energy vision without knowing whether you will achieve it or not. A client once told me that he will create a vision only if he knows for certain that he can reach it. This is not an attitude that promotes energetic behavior. Achievements can be most satisfying when you are not sure that you can accomplish something and manage to do it anyway. If you only agree to do what you *know* you can do, then you are playing it safe; and safe will not increase your energy—rather, it will subtract from it.

Creating a high-energy vision involves listening to and trusting your instincts. If you know in your heart that it's time to change the way you treat yourself, then use this knowledge as motivation to create the vision that will lead you to the next phase of your career. If you follow your instincts (your true inner voice and not a fleeting emotion) you will be led in the right direction.

STEPS FOR CREATING YOUR HIGH-ENERGY VISION

Here are five steps for taping into your instincts to create your vision:

1. Make time to think

2. Ask yourself what you want

3. Write down what you want

4. Organize your thoughts

5. Finalize your vision

Now, let's go through each one separately:

1. Make time to think

A clear picture of yourself as a high-energy person cannot come to you unless you create a space in your mind to think about it. This space is what will allow you to get in touch with yourself and your priorities. This space is where you will create your vision.

One of the main reasons your energy is lacking is because you are "busy," so you have to take care that being busy does not keep you from making time to work on your vision. Time to create your vision will not be given to you—you have to take it. This does not mean that you have to allocate days or weeks of thought to nothing else but your vision; but regularly taking an hour here and half an hour there will make a tremendous difference.

Ask yourself, "When will I make time to think about what I want?" Notice that I am not telling you to ask yourself *whether* you will *find* time, but rather *when* you will *make* the time. It is essential to be assertive with yourself.

> Note: The time you are making in your schedule now will continue to be used as your high-energy journey progresses. Currently, you will use this time to create your vision. Next, you will use it to create a high-energy plan to make your vision come to life. Finally, you will use the time to implement your plan. If you are reading this section and saying to yourself that you cannot make the time, I would like you to reconsider. If I said to you that I would give you a million dollars to create your vision this week, I bet that you would find the time to do it. You would do whatever was necessary because you wanted the money. My hope is that you want, with the same purpose and intensity, to have energy. Surely, your health is at least as important to you as a million dollars—likely, it's worth far, far more. Make the time. This time will be important to reaching your goal of feeling great every day. This time is vital for your success.

Knowing your body and your schedule, when is the best time for you to think? If you get your best thinking done earlier in the day, then get up fifteen minutes early to work on your vision. I had a client who said she had great intentions of thinking in the morning, but somehow time slipped away from her. In response,

I suggested a timer—when it was time for her to think about her vision, the timer reminded her to stop whatever she was doing, so that she could get her thinking done. You may be laughing as you read this, but whatever works, works. Find the best time for you, and tap into this time regularly, using a tool such as a timer if you need one.

Ask your family to support you and hold you accountable to your plan to make time for thinking. It's easy to say before you go to bed that you will get up early the next day; but it's a different story when the alarm rings, and you feel like rolling over and going back to sleep. Ask family members to make sure you get up. Tell them to ignore your requests for them to go away. If you need help, ask for it. If you don't live with someone who can make sure you wake up, make a point of reminding yourself, as soon as that alarm goes off, *why* you are getting up early in the first place. It's because having high energy is important to you—important enough to miss fifteen minutes of sleep in order to start the process of getting it. Tell yourself that if you go back to sleep, you will feel worse later on because you did not make time to think about your future. If you don't attack it at the first opportunity you have, the task of creating your vision will hang over your head all day. You will feel bad that you did not work on it. Keeping this in mind, isn't it easier to just get up and do it? You will feel much better if you do.

If you are not a morning person, what time is good for you? Lunchtime? After work? The weekends? Find a time that is right for you.

Once you have made the time, find a quiet place. Ask your family (or supportive co-workers) not to disturb you. Sit down and take deep breaths, as many as you need to instill a sense of calmness. Your mind will want to wander, but you must bring yourself back. Remind yourself why you are doing this. You want to make changes in your energy level. Focus on the importance of this to your career, and channel your thoughts in this direction.

2. Ask yourself what you want

When you are in a quiet place, close your eyes. Let your imagination take over. Get in touch with what you really want and what is important to you.

Do this by asking yourself the following questions:

- If it was possible to feel great at work every day and impossible to fail, what would be different in my career?
- What type of job would I have?
- What would I be responsible for?
- What type of boss/co-workers/team would I have?
- What kind of hours would I work?
- What type of company would I work for?
- What sort of culture would the company have?
- What city would I live in?
- How much money would I make?
- How would I handle stress, my workload, and deadlines?
- How would I successfully be balancing work and life?
- How much would I weigh?
- What foods would I be eating? (Or not eating?)
- What type of exercise would I be doing?
- How many hours of sleep would I get?

There are no right or wrong answers to these questions. The answers are what is true for you—not what someone else wants for you, but what is truly in your heart. Listen to yourself, and your answers will be the perfect ones for you.

Be careful not to screen yourself or talk yourself out of your answers. Whether you have tried in the past (and failed) to obtain high energy in your career does not matter. You are trying *now*, and this is what counts. In addition, don't let past mistakes or choices cloud your answers. You may have been making decisions in your career that have limited your energy, but this does not mean that it's too late for you to turn things around.

> Whatever the answers, let them come to you; and accept them, whatever they may be. Knowledge is power. It's better to know than to not know.

If you have been asking yourself these questions and still can't figure out what you want, start thinking about what you *don't* want. You'll often find that the opposite is what you want. "What type of job would I have?" Think about jobs you have had that you did not like. What, specifically, did not work for you? What would you like to be different next time? Your answers will give you clues as to what you really want to be doing. "What would I be eating?" Begin with what you've been eating that you know is not good for your body. This knowledge will lead to better food choices.

Discovering what you want can be tricky. Maybe you have not asked yourself these questions in many years, and you are unsure how to answer them. Maybe you used to know, long ago, what you wanted or needed to do to feel better again, but have forgotten. Maybe you know the answers but are afraid of them, because acting on them will be difficult. Meditation, prayer, and keeping a journal are good techniques to help you gain clarity regarding these answers.

Adopt the premise that your career wishes can and will be fulfilled. If you tell yourself that you will be successful, you will be.

---

3. Write down what you want

Once you have seriously thought about these questions, it is time to get your answers down on paper (or on your computer screen). You can answer the questions I have provided previously; or come up with questions of your own. Your bigger goal is to take your answers and turn them into a description (a vision) of you as a healthy, high-energy individual.

First, make a list of what you want. Write without editing yourself. Don't worry about the order of the list for now—you will organize it later.

Here's an example of a list you could create:

If I had my way …

1.   I would have a career that energized me.

2.   I would not worry about money, because I would have a career that pays me well.

3. I would wake up and look forward to the day.

4. I would be in great shape.

5. I would eat meals that are delicious and nutritious.

6. I would feel calm even when everyone around me was stressed.

7. I would work no more than eight hours a day.

8. I would work in a location with plenty of sunshine.

9. I would commute no more than a half hour each way.

10. I would work on projects that made a real difference.

11. I would have great relationships with my boss, co-workers, and staff.

12. I would work with supportive people.

13. I would work in a company that cared about its people.

Now, make a list of your own. If I had my way, and I had a high-energy career:

1. Item #1—I would:

2. Item #2—I would:

3. Item #3—I would:

4. Item #4—I would:

5. Item #5—I would:

6. Item #6—I would:

7. Item #7—I would:

8. Item #8—I would:

9. Item #9—I would:

10. Item #10—I would:

Do you think your list (or the sample one I created) contains a series of impossible dreams? Don't let negative thinking get in the way. Keep listing items. Keep listening to your heart as you write. Keep writing down what is true for you. Keep asking yourself, "What do I want?" Try your best to block out competing thoughts as you write. If you want to give yourself the greatest chance of creating a vision that will guide you through the next phase of your career, stop distracting yourself with negativity. The words you write down—*your* words—are important. They are the beginning of a vision that will empower you and give you something to look forward to.

4. Organize your thoughts

Writing without boundaries has allowed you to get all of your desires down in concrete form. Your next task is to format your list so that it makes more sense and is easy for you to follow. Let's use the list from the previous section. Below, I have arranged the items in order of importance:

If I had my way ...

1. I would have a career that energized me.

2. I would work in a company that cared about its people.

3. I would work on projects that made a real difference.

4. I would not worry about money, because I would have a career that pays me well.

5. I would have great relationships with my boss, co-workers, and staff.

6. I would work with supportive people.

7. I would work in a location with plenty of sunshine.

8. I would work no more than eight hours a day.

9. I would commute no more than a half hour each way.

10. I would be in great shape.

11. I would eat meals that are delicious and nutritious.

12. I would feel calm when everyone around me was stressed.

13. I would wake up every morning and look forward to the day.

Now, put your list in order of importance to you. If I had my way, I would:

1. Item #1—I would:

2. Item #2—I would:

3. Item #3—I would:

4. Item #4—I would:

5. Item #5—I would:

6. Item #6—I would:

7. Item #7—I would:

8. Item #8—I would:

9. Item #9—I would:

10. Item #10—I would:

5. Finalize your vision

Now, transform this list into your high-energy vision—a description of everything that is important to you. Here's the finalized vision from the sample list I have provided:

> *I will have a career that energizes me. I will work for a company that cares about its people and be responsible for projects that make a difference. I will be paid well for my contributions. I will have a great relationship with my boss, co-workers, and staff, and work with supportive people. I will work in a location with plenty of sunshine, for no more than eight hours a day. I will commute no more than a half hour each way. I will be in great shape. I will eat meals that are delicious and nutritious. I will feel calm when everyone around me is stressed and I will wake up every morning looking forward to the day.*

Now, using your list, create your own vision:

Put your vision here.

Are you still wondering if your vision can come true? If so, remember that it can, as long as you were listening intently to yourself during the vision creating process.

Your vision came from your heart, so believe it is perfect and obtainable.

Will your vision change over time? Possibly. But whether it changes or not, what you have created today is right for the current stage of your career. Your vision does not have to be written in stone. It can be changed as you progress. Today's vision is a starting point. If you find that, for whatever reason, it really does not work, you can always tweak it. For the purpose of moving forward, work with what you have now.

LOOKING AT YOUR HIGH-ENERGY VISION EVERY DAY

Once your vision has been created, you will want to keep it alive. Look at your vision every morning so you can start your day with focus. Look at your vision every evening, so that it stays with you in your dreams. Looking at and contemplating your vision plays a large role in making it real.

If you create your vision and put it away, your words will have no value. What you can't see will soon be forgotten. But when you look at your vision regularly, it will gradually become a part of who you are. As discussed at the beginning of this section, all goals are reached in the mind first. When you can see yourself achieving the vision you created, it will make it easier to achieve in reality.

Step 4:
Build Your High-Energy
Career Success Plan

There really is no mystery to reaching goals. You listen to what is in your heart (which is your vision) and then you create a plan to make your vision happen. Once you have your plan—which details how you will make your vision real—you work on the actions in your plan on a consistent basis. Then you reach your goals. That's it.

Many clients have asked me whether I think they will be successful in reaching their goals. My answer is yes—*if* they do the work. If you are making time for your goals, I believe that you will reach them. If you are not working on your goals regularly, then they will be more difficult to achieve. If you are thinking about and working on your goals every day, success will be yours.

Having a plan is vital to your success. With a plan, a career filled with energy will be far easier to achieve. Without a plan, you will be working far harder than you have to.

The trick is to be clear about the steps that are necessary to ensure your success. The more specific you can be in describing your steps, the better. Figuring out in detail what steps you will take—and when you will take them—is the foundation of your plan.

Another reason to create a plan is that it will prevent your high-energy goal from becoming overwhelming. The temptation to feel overwhelmed is normal. You are, after all, about to embark on a change. The structure of your plan will give you comfort and help you with your transition.

HOW TO CREATE YOUR PLAN

There are two main components of your high-energy career success plan:

1. What you want (your vision)

2. How you will get there (the specific steps—or mini-goals—you need to carry out along the way)

You will know that you have a good, workable plan when you have taken your vision and divided it into specific steps that are clear and easy to follow. The length of your plan is not important. What matters is you have a document that you can study and follow every day.

Why do your steps have to be specific? Without specific steps, you will be floating without direction. In addition, these steps are an excellent way to measure how close you are to achieving your goals.

Let's go through how the two main components of your high-energy career success plan work. I will use the high-energy vision from the last chapter to show you. Follow along with the vision example I put together, and then go through the exercise using the vision that you developed for yourself. Here again is the example I created:

> *I will have a career that energizes me. I will work for a company that cares about its people and be responsible for projects that make a difference. I will be paid well for my contributions. I will have a great relationship with my boss, co-workers, and staff, and work with supportive people. I will work in a location with plenty of sunshine, for no more than eight hours a day. I will commute no more than a half hour each way. I will be in great shape. I will eat meals that are delicious and nutritious. I will feel calm when everyone around me is stressed and I will wake up every morning looking forward to the day.*

Let's take this vision and break it into individual statements and specific steps.

I will have a career that energizes me. (Vision Statement #1)

Specific steps might be:

- I will decide to have a career that energizes me.

- I will tell myself every day that it's possible to have a career that energizes me.

- I will make a list of what I would be doing differently if I had a career that energized me.

- I will create a description of where I want my career to be in a year, in three years, in five years, and farther into the future. I will decide that this description will come true.

- I will list what I like about my career.

- I will list what I don't like.

- I will list what I can eliminate.

- I will list what I can delegate.

- I will list the tasks that give me energy.

- I will list the tasks that rob me of my energy.

- I will list ways to bring more spirituality into my career.

- I will create a description of what an energizing career means to me. I will include what I would be doing and not doing, where I would be working, and everything else that would be relevant to such a career.

- I will compare this description to my current career.

- If the description is a match, I will list ways in which I can bring more energy to my present job. If the description is not a match, I will make a list of companies that I would like to work for that do match this description.

- I will read a newspaper every day and one magazine each week, looking for companies that inspire me. I will either decide that I want to work for one of these companies, or list ways in which I will incorporate what makes these companies successful into my current role.

- I will talk to one person each week who has a career that he or she loves and ask how he or she got there.

I will work for a company that cares about its people. (Vision Statement #2)

Specific steps might be:

- I will decide that I want to work for a company that cares about its people.

- I will assess whether my current company cares about its people.

- I will assess whether there are departments within my company that care about their people.

- I will assess whether my company/department is open to caring about its people. If it is, I will list ways that in which it can be more caring.

- If my company/department is really open to being more caring, I will create a plan to make the items on my list happen.

- If where I am working now does not seem to care for its people, then I will research companies that *do*. I will use the Internet, newspapers, magazines, people I know, and even people I don't know to help me find the type of company I am looking for.

- I will list ways in which I can be more caring.

I will be responsible for projects that make a difference. (Vision Statement #3)

Specific steps might be:

- I will decide that the projects I work on will make a difference.

- I will make a list of the projects I am currently working on.

- I will assess whether or not the projects I am working on are making a difference.

- If they are not, I will write down ways in which they can do so in the future.

- I will make a list of different projects I might want to work on.

- I will make an appointment with my boss to request that I be assigned to some of these projects.

- I will do my research and be able to tell my boss how he/she and the company will benefit if my request is granted.

I will be paid well for my contributions. (Vision Statement #4)

Specific steps might be:

- I will decide that I will be paid well for my contributions.

- I will be making at least $_____ per year by the end of this year.

- I will use the Internet to research what my position is worth.

- I will contact associations related to my industry to see what salaries are being paid for positions equivalent to mine.

- I will compare what I want to be paid with what the marketplace is paying.

- I will decide whether I want to find a new job paying the salary I want, or to request a raise at my current employer.

- If I want to stay where I am, I will assemble a list of what I have contributed to the company, so I have evidence of why I should be making more money.

- If I need to go back to school to update my skills so that I can earn more money, I will research what schools are available, what they cost, and whether or not they are worth the investment.

- I will research different companies to find out which of them pay their employees well.

- I will decide whether I want to work for one of these companies.

I will have great relationships with my boss, co-workers, and staff. (Vision Statement #5)

Specific steps might be:

- I will decide to have great relationships with my boss, co-workers, and staff.

- I will be nice to everyone I work with.

- I will say hello to everyone I see at the beginning of the day and good-night to them at the end.

- I will ask the people I work with about their interests outside of work. I will make time to listen to the answer, remember what they said, and ask them about their interests from time to time.

- I will no longer gossip.

- If I have a conflict with someone I work with, I will talk to this person directly.

- I will make an appointment this week with _____, so that I can create a better working relationship with him/her.

- I will listen better.

- I will communicate better.

- I will arrange weekly meetings with my boss, co-workers, and staff, so that I can stay connected and updated.

- I will do what I say I will do.

- I will return phone calls and e-mails in a timely fashion.

- I will have lunch with one person each week with whom I normally would not socialize.

- I will push myself away from my desk, rely less on e-mail, and talk to more people face-to-face.

I will work with supportive people. (Vision Statement #6)

Specific steps might be:

- I will decide to work with supportive people.

- I will list ways in which I can become more supportive.

- I will do at least one thing on this list each week.

- I will listen better.

- I will communicate better.

- I will do what I say I will do.

- I will ask my boss, co-workers, and staff if they need help with projects they are working on.

- I will let go of my expectations of how the people I work with should be and accept who they are.

<u>I will work in a location with plenty of sunshine. (Vision Statement #7)</u>

Specific steps might be:

- I will decide to work in a location with plenty of sunshine.
- I will assess whether I am working in a state or country where the sun shines regularly.
- I will assess whether I am working for a company that lets the sun shine into its buildings.
- I will assess whether I am getting outside enough during the day to see the sun.
- If there is space available that is sunnier, I will request to sit there.
- If sunlight is not possible, I will look into purchasing a sun lamp.

<u>I will work for no more than eight hours a day. (Vision Statement #8)</u>

Specific steps might be:

- I will decide to work for no more than eight hours a day.
- I will list what I am responsible for and note how long I believe each task takes.
- I will create a week-long journal in which I will carefully note where I am actually spending my time.
- At the end of the week, I will look at my journal and determine whether I am using my time wisely or not.
- If I am not using my time wisely, I will list distractions and ways in which I am not as efficient as I'd like to be.
- I will list ways in which I can be more productive.
- If I am using my time wisely, I will make a list of tasks I may be able to eliminate, delegate, or streamline.
- I will make a promise to myself that I will no work longer than eight hours a day.
- I will list ways in which I can fulfill this promise.
- If my company demands that I work more than eight hours a day, I will decide whether or not I want to continue working for this company.

- I will research companies that believe in a healthy work/life balance.
- I will decide whether I want to work for one of these companies.

I will commute no more than a half hour each way. (Vision Statement #9)

Specific steps might be:

- I will decide that my commute will be less than a half-hour each way.
- I will time my regular commute in order to see how long it takes.
- I will research alternative routes or public transportation which may shorten my commute.
- I will research whether moving closer to my company is an option.
- I will try commuting at different times of the morning and evening in order to find a time that is less crowded.
- I will inquire whether I can telecommute for some portion of the week.
- I will request to telecommute. I will tell my boss how he/she and the company stand to benefit if my request is honored.
- If my commute is longer than a half hour each way, I will make a list of companies in my industry that are closer to my home.
- I will decide whether I want to work for one of these companies.

I will be in great shape. (Vision Statement #10)

Specific steps might be:

- I will decide that my body will be in great shape.
- I will set a goal of losing ten pounds over the next ninety days.
- I will exercise at least three days per week.
- I will decide when is the best time for me to fit a workout into my schedule.
- I will either get up earlier to work out or take my gym clothes to the office so that I can work out during lunch or after work.
- I will decide how I like to exercise, whether it is in a gym, as part of a sports team, or walking/jogging/cycling outside.

- I will join a gym or hire a personal trainer.
- I will join a sports team or a walking club.
- I will take a yoga class.
- I will run a marathon.
- I will stretch at my desk.
- I will purchase reasonably-priced exercise equipment for my home.
- I will identify three people who might like to work out with me.
- I will ask these three people this week if they would like to join me.
- I will find someone to support me and hold me accountable to my decision to get my body into great shape.
- I will sleep for eight hours per night so that my body can rest and recover properly.

<u>I will eat meals that are delicious and nutritious. (Vision Statement #11)</u>

Specific steps might be:

- I will decide to eat meals that are delicious and nutritious.
- I will plan what I will eat at work.
- I will stick to my plan.
- I will bring healthy snacks into the office with me every day.
- I will stay away from foods that are processed, have high sugar content, or are fried.
- I will stay away from vending machines.
- I will make the best choices for my body one meal at a time.
- I will eat a salad for lunch or with my meal.
- I will say no to the cookies and cake that are in the kitchen and conference room.
- I will not give in to food cravings.
- I will choose foods that come from the land rather than those processed by man.

- I will read the ingredients of foods and choose to eat only foods with ingredients I know are healthy for me.

- I will drink water instead of soda.

- I will not have more than two cups of coffee per day.

<u>I will feel calm when everyone around me is stressed. (Vision Statement #12)</u>

Specific steps might be:

- I will decide to feel calm when everyone around me is stressed.

- I will take deep breaths before speaking or acting.

- I will tell myself that no matter what the crisis at hand may be, I will find a way to work through it. I will remind myself of past crises and how well I handled them.

- I will refrain from sugar and caffeine, which make me jittery.

- I will take breaks during the day.

- I will keep calming items on my desk.

- I will listen to calming music during the day.

<u>I will wake up every morning looking forward to the day. (Vision Statement #13)</u>

Specific steps might be:

- I will decide to wake up every morning looking forward to the day.

- I will decide to be more passionate about my career.

- I will meditate every morning.

- I will plan my day the night before, so that I wake up focused.

- In the evenings, I will lay out my clothes and other items I will need for the following day, so that I can get up, get ready, and leave the house without stress and in an organized manner.

- I will make a list of what I love about my career.

- I will look at this list every morning.

- I will read and/or listen to motivational materials on the way to and from work.

- I will tell myself each morning that the day is going to be a great one.

Now it's your turn. Divide your vision into individual statements. Then list the specific steps you will take to make each statement happen.

List the steps that you know you absolutely need to do. You can always add more steps later.

Write your vision here.

Vision Statement #1: _____

- Specific Step #1:
- Specific Step #2:
- Specific Step #3:
- Specific Step #4:
- Specific Step #5:

Vision Statement #2: _____

- Specific Step #1:
- Specific Step #2:
- Specific Step #3:
- Specific Step #4:
- Specific Step #5:

Vision Statement #3: _____

- Specific Step #1:
- Specific Step #2:
- Specific Step #3:
- Specific Step #4:
- Specific Step #5:

Vision Statement #4: _____

- Specific Step #1:
- Specific Step #2:
- Specific Step #3:
- Specific Step #4:
- Specific Step #5:

Vision Statement #5: _____

- Specific Step #1:
- Specific Step #2:
- Specific Step #3:
- Specific Step #4:
- Specific Step #5:

Vision Statement #6: _____

- Specific Step #1:
- Specific Step #2:
- Specific Step #3:
- Specific Step #4:
- Specific Step #5:

Vision Statement #7: _____

- Specific Step #1:
- Specific Step #2:
- Specific Step #3:
- Specific Step #4:
- Specific Step #5:

Vision Statement #8: _____

- Specific Step #1:
- Specific Step #2:
- Specific Step #3:
- Specific Step #4:
- Specific Step #5:

Vision Statement #9: _____

- Specific Step #1:
- Specific Step #2:
- Specific Step #3:
- Specific Step #4:
- Specific Step #5:

Vision Statement #10: _____

- Specific Step #1:
- Specific Step #2:
- Specific Step #3:
- Specific Step #4:
- Specific Step #5:

CHOOSE WHERE TO BEGIN

Next, decide which statement and steps you will begin with.

> Choose the statement and steps you consider to be the most important to implement first. Start where your instincts tell you to begin.

For example, from my own sample lists, I choose working on projects that make a difference as my first goal. (Vision Statement #3)

Here's that statement again:

I will be responsible for projects that make a difference.

- I will decide that the projects I work on will make a difference.
- I will make a list of the projects I am currently working on.
- I will assess whether or not the projects I am working on are making a difference.
- If they are not, I will write down ways in which they can do so in the future.
- I will make a list of different projects I might want to work on.
- I will make an appointment with my boss to request that I be assigned to some of these projects.
- I will do my research and be able to tell my boss how he/she and the company will benefit if my request is granted.

Now, it's your turn.

Select the statement that you believe will give you the largest amount of energy. Write it down and list its steps here.

Most Important Vision Statement: _____

- Specific Step #1:
- Specific Step #2:
- Specific Step #3:
- Specific Step #4:
- Specific Step #5:

Now, go through your entire list and prioritize the statements. Choose the statements that you believe you need to do first, second, third, and so on. Prioritizing the statements gives you the order in which you will attack each one. Again, trust your instincts when prioritizing. There is no right or wrong place to begin—there is only what feels right to you.

Vision Statement Priority #2: _____

- Specific Step #1:
- Specific Step #2:
- Specific Step #3:
- Specific Step #4:
- Specific Step #5:

Vision Statement Priority #3: _____

- Specific Step #1:
- Specific Step #2:
- Specific Step #3:
- Specific Step #4:
- Specific Step #5:

Vision Statement Priority #4: _____

- Specific Step #1:
- Specific Step #2:
- Specific Step #3:
- Specific Step #4:
- Specific Step #5:

Vision Statement Priority #5: _____

- Specific Step #1:
- Specific Step #2:
- Specific Step #3:
- Specific Step #4:
- Specific Step #5:

Vision Statement Priority #6: _____

- Specific Step #1:
- Specific Step #2:

- Specific Step #3:
- Specific Step #4:
- Specific Step #5:

Vision Statement Priority #7: _____

- Specific Step #1:
- Specific Step #2:
- Specific Step #3:
- Specific Step #4:
- Specific Step #5:

Vision Statement Priority #8: _____

- Specific Step #1:
- Specific Step #2:
- Specific Step #3:
- Specific Step #4:
- Specific Step #5:

Vision Statement Priority #9: _____

- Specific Step #1:
- Specific Step #2:
- Specific Step #3:
- Specific Step #4:
- Specific Step #5:

Vision Statement Priority #10: _____

- Specific Step #1:
- Specific Step #2:
- Specific Step #3:
- Specific Step #4:
- Specific Step #5:

Congratulations! You have just created a detailed plan of the steps that will lead you to the realization of your vision. This is a major achievement.

Note: If you are still a bit unsure of what all of your steps are, work with what you have created up to this point. One of your steps can be to find out what steps you are missing. Move forward anyway with your plan, even if all of your steps haven't been filled in yet. As you go through the process of bringing more energy into your career, the steps for doing so will become clearer.

Please also note that a plan does not have to be a complicated document. All it needs to contain is what you want and the steps you will take to make what you want a reality. Once you have all your steps listed, you have the luxury of choosing which one you would like to work on first. Once you have chosen a starting point, you progress through the steps *one by one*, until there are no more steps to take. When you are out of steps, you can celebrate, because you have arrived at your destination.

COMMIT TO YOUR PLAN

Just as you decided to get healthy, it's important to decide that you will make your high-energy success plan happen. You do this by simply saying, "I will commit to my plan and my desire to feel energized."

You might be able to think of dozens of reasons not to commit to your plan now. Maybe you are afraid that the work you are about to do will not really make a difference. Maybe you are concerned that your co-workers will think you are odd when you change your usual routine. Maybe you are worried that your newfound energy will cause you to stick out from the crowd more than you're accustomed to. You have too much at stake to let your doubts stop you.

Keep in mind that your plan is a sort of game. Of course, you want to win the game—but just being on the court is important in itself. As long as you are playing, and you are trying your best to get energized, you can win.

Yet, the ball cannot be thrown to you unless you are on the field to catch it. You would of course be more comfortable knowing ahead of time that you will be successful; or that every single moment you spend on court will be fun and worthwhile. Unfortunately, you will not get that guarantee up front. Your energy level will increase when you put yourself on the field and accept what happens there—mistakes and all. Accept what may happen, yet stand strong in your commitment to what you want to happen. When you do, you will be taking a tremendous positive step in the right direction.

Step 5:
Take Action

When you are taking action, you are carrying out the steps in your plan with purpose and power. You are "in the zone" and believe that anything is possible. You feel great. You have faith that your steps will lead to high energy. And you are right.

Action is essential to your success. Therefore, every day, you must work on your plan for it to happen.

> Do a little bit every day. Your efforts, whether big or small, will all add up and make a remarkable difference in the results you achieve.

OPEN YOUR CALENDAR

One of the best ways to keep your momentum going is having the steps in your plan written into your calendar. Your calendar is an essential tool for helping you reach your high-energy goal.

Having a calendar will help determine whether you are victorious or not. If you don't feel like taking a step, your calendar can help you get motivated and stay on track. If you don't remember what your next step is, your calendar will remind you what to work on. If your steps are written into your calendar, there is a higher probability that you can quickly check them off your list, because what you need to do is in front of you. If your steps are not in your calendar, they probably will not get done, because you may forget what you need to do.

Note: Your calendar can be paper or electronic. The format is not important. What is important is choosing a method you like and will use consistently.

Your calendar is your friend. Begin your friendship by opening your calendar and entering the steps from your plan into it. Start with the vision statement and steps that you deemed most important to you. For example, in the last chapter, I used my own example of Vision Statement #3—working on projects that make a difference—as the step that I believed would provide me with the most energy. Let me show you how you could put that statement into a calendar.

Now, let's say that it's Sunday evening, and I am deciding what to work on over the next couple of weeks. Here is an illustration of how I would plan my time and specifically what I would put into my calendar:

- I will decide that the projects I work on will make a difference.

  (I will do that now.)

- I will make a list of the projects I am currently working on.

  (I will do that tomorrow morning from 8:00 AM to 9:00 AM.)

- I will assess whether the projects I am working on are making a difference.

  (I will do that on Tuesday & Wednesday mornings this week from 8:00 AM to 9:00 AM.)

- If they are not, I will write down ways in which they can do so in the future.

  (I will do that on Thursday and Friday mornings of this week from 8:00 AM to 9:00 AM.)

- I will make a list of different projects I might want to work on.

  (I will do that next Saturday & Sunday mornings from 9:00 AM to 11:00 AM. I will also go over my list the following Monday morning from 8:00 AM to 9:00 AM.)

- I will make an appointment with my boss to request that I be assigned to some of these projects.

  (I will arrange this appointment for the Monday two weeks from tomorrow.)

- I will do my research and be able to tell my boss how he/she and the company will benefit if my request is granted.

  (I will do that next week on Tuesday through Friday from 8:00 AM to 9:00 AM.)

Why did I choose only mornings in this example? Most people do their best thinking and planning in the morning. In addition, once your workday gets started, it's harder to switch gears and do something for yourself. Nevertheless, choose the best times to work on your steps according to your own preferences.

Now, it's your turn.

Plan your time. Put each step and the time chosen for each step into your calendar one by one. Again, begin with the vision statement and steps that you deem the most important to you. You can stop where you are (and get to your other vision statements later) or do the same for each remaining vision statement and its corresponding steps now. Remember that your goal is high energy, not overwhelm, so whichever steps you feel comfortable entering into your calendar at this time are the perfect steps to enter.

MAKE YOUR PLAN REAL

Making your high-energy career success plan a reality happens when you are moving forward on a daily basis, while occasionally pausing to review, regroup, and prepare for the next steps you plan to work on.

The process of implementing your plan can be divided into three components:

1. Taking action
2. Reviewing the steps you have taken
3. Preparing for your next steps

Let's go through each one.

1. Taking action

Goals are reached when you are actively working on them. As I stated earlier, mapping out what you are going to do—and then doing it—is your recipe for success.

If you were to complete one step from your plan every day, you will have taken thirty steps at the end of the month and 365 steps by the end of the year. These small steps can take you a long way. Small steps add up to big ones. Your plan is going to be achieved one step at a time.

2. Reviewing the steps you have taken

On some days, you will do everything you have planned, and some days you will not. Don't let this discourage you.

Sometimes you may feel that you are not progressing as fast as you'd like. At these times, remember that despite your best intentions, you are not a machine. Your job may get extra busy from time to time, and unexpected things may crop up that demand your immediate attention. Of course, you must take care of these things. You also need to take time out for rest if you are feeling exhausted. It is OK to stray slightly from your plan every once in a while—but if you have begun to neglect it completely, it is important to note why. Are you afraid to take the next step? Are you truly committed to having high energy? Do you need to revisit your vision or the steps in your plan and revise them? It is fine to take a step back, or a break, if that's what you think you need to move forward again.

If you do decide to take a break, still take the time to ask yourself:
Am I doing what I promised myself I would?
Do I need to tweak my vision?
Do I need to readjust the priority of my steps?
Do I need to rearrange the scheduling of my steps in my calendar?

Part of the journey of becoming a high-energy individual is learning what works and what doesn't. This is a normal part of the process. Review and reassess as much as you feel is necessary.

3. Preparing for your next steps

Sit down with your calendar on Sunday evenings. Go over your plan and the steps you will be working on during the coming week. Write down in your calendar specifically when you will be working on each step. Every day, review your calendar. This routine will keep you on top of both your weekly and daily tasks.

Don't forget to look at your high-energy vision every day too. When you can see your future, you will find that it will arrive quicker than you think.

KEEP THE FUTURE IN MIND

In order for the future to arrive quickly, you may have to make a few changes on your journey. Ask yourself if there is anything that you have to let go of—or improve—to ensure that your high-energy career success plan succeeds.

> Your future cannot materialize if the present is in the way.

For example:

- Do you need to stop telling yourself that you don't have enough time to work on your plan?
- Do you need to prioritize better?
- Do you need to create a new routine that will keep you focused?
- Do you need to ask for help?

What follows are some tips that will help you overcome these obstacles.

MANAGE YOUR TIME

Like most people today, you are probably extremely busy—and you are certainly not alone in this. But do not use being busy as an excuse. It's essential to work on your plan despite what is happening around you. If you do not make time to create high energy, it will not magically occur on its own. Is high energy important to you? If the answer is yes, then you will have to make time available for it to happen.

Consider your current job. What is occupying most of your time? Can you eliminate some of those tasks? Can you delegate them? Can you streamline your methods of doing them? Can you postpone them? If a way exists to free up some of your time, you owe it to yourself to find it.

The steps in your plan will take time to implement. So, can you get up earlier in the morning to work on them? Can you do one step during lunch? Can you implement one step in the evening? Can you do some planning during your commute? Can you arrange your evenings differently, to allow yourself to prepare effectively for the next day?

Your workload will always be there. Will your health?

SELECT YOUR PRIORITIES

There will always be something on your list of things to do. Do what you can. Accomplishing tasks helps reduce stress and anxiety, but you should avoid expecting to do too many of them simultaneously. You are better off under-promising and over-delivering than taking on too much at one time. You don't have to implement your entire plan today. Your plan will unfold over time. Do your best and be proud of yourself for doing so.

Let go of what you *should* do, or *could* do. Instead, focus on what you *want* to do and accomplish. You *want* to get healthy and feel great at work. This is your objective. As you review your plan and schedule steps into your calendar, keep asking yourself:

- What is the most important thing for me to do today, this week, etc.?
- What steps will get me closer to my high-energy goal?
- What needs to be done right away?
- What can be done quickly and easily?

- How can I best use my time?
- How can I work intelligently, as opposed to simply working hard?

Adjust your plan as necessary. Customize it according to your own needs and desires. You can implement it in any way that you like. Select the steps you want to work on, and work on them. This is how you will reach your ultimate goal of having more energy.

When your career gets hectic—and sometimes it will—don't forget about your mental and physical health. This must be a priority. If you do not put yourself first, you will not have much energy left for anything else. You cannot feel great in your career unless you take care of yourself first.

CHANGE YOUR ROUTINE

Do you wake up the same time every day? Do you take the same route to work, eat the same breakfast, see the same people, work on the same projects, and spend your evenings in the same way every day? Do you do all this while eagerly counting the days remaining until the weekend?

If you have answered yes to most of these questions, you may be in a rut which is contributing to your low energy level. If so, you can do something about it.

Of course, routines are not bad things in themselves. They can reduce stress and feelings of being overwhelmed. If you had to think about every little detail of your day and how to go about it, you probably wouldn't function very well.

However, you want to eliminate routines that are affecting your energy level. Do you have a cup of coffee with two tablespoons of sugar and a doughnut every morning at 8:00 AM? This is a routine that will bring your energy level up quickly—and crash it just as quickly about an hour later. Do you have a chocolate bar every day at 3:00 PM? This is also a routine that will hurt your energy level and contribute to weight gain. Do you continually work fourteen-hour days and get little rest on the weekends? This is a routine that will burn you out.

How about creating healthy new routines? Why not eat egg whites for breakfast instead of a doughnut? Or drinking water instead of coffee? Decide what new healthy routines you will incorporate into your days from now on, and start doing them. And of course, don't forget to put your new routines into your calendar.

GET SUPPORT

I meet many people who are unhappy with their careers, but they hesitate to ask for help. I believe that this is because they feel embarrassed about feeling unable to tackle their career challenges by themselves. Humans, however, are not meant to handle most problems by themselves. Above all, we are social beings. We need one another to help us reach our goals, especially when we feel tired and our energy levels are low.

You are about to embark on a journey that will change for the better how you view yourself and conduct your career. Why would you want to make this change alone? Your road to high energy will be harder and longer if you take it by yourself. Your chances of success will also drop substantially.

Asking for help does not mean that you will need assistance for the rest of your career. But right now, you do. After all, isn't that why you chose to read this book? Pay no mind to worries about what people might think of you. Everyone needs help from time to time. Now, it's your turn. Somewhere down the road, you may help the people who helped you.

It's OK to ask for help. If a dear friend or family member asked you to help them, wouldn't you say yes? Why wouldn't they say yes to you? One thing you can say for certain is that they definitely will not be able to say yes if you do not ask them.

Don't wait. Ask for help as soon as you need it.

MOVE FORWARD NO MATTER WHAT

I've seen many people on the brink of success fail because they stopped right before they reached their goal.

> Those who are successful in attaining high energy are those who do not give up.

Your plan is a work in progress. As such, you may get sidetracked from time to time. This is OK—such important processes cannot always be smooth ones. If you get frustrated every once in a while, remember that you are not alone.

You are not perfect. You will occasionally make mistakes. You may even fall back into your old ways from time to time. Be patient with yourself and keep returning to your high-energy career success plan to keep you on track.

Move forward no matter what. You will have good days and bad days—everyone does. Nevertheless, try to move yourself forward even if you do not feel like it on a particular day. Take one step every day whether you believe it will make a difference or not. Movement will help make your high-energy goals a reality.

Step 6:
Arrive At Your Destination

The premise of this book is that you will succeed. You *will* reach your high-energy goal.

Sooner or later, if you follow the steps in this book, you will arrive at your destination. When you do, I would like to be the first to congratulate you! And don't forget to applaud *yourself* for your hard work and effort.

ACKNOWLEDGEMENT

Arriving at your destination is an important part of your high-energy career success plan because it allows you to let in the great job you have done in reaching your goal. It's also a time to recognize your accomplishments. When you reach your goal, you can acknowledge yourself for having gone after what you wanted and succeeding. Not only will your journey have built character, it will have made you a happier and healthier person.

ENJOY THE NEW HIGH-ENERGY YOU

Do you think you will feel different after you carry out your plan? You should because you will. You will be doing things that you were not doing before. Maybe you will go after that promotion you wanted—or that new job. Maybe you will buy yourself a new wardrobe because your new eating and exercising habits will have reshaped your body. Maybe you will enjoy the company of your friends and family more because you feel better.

You will be enjoying your new life tremendously. And you will deserve it.

KEEP THE MOMENTUM GOING

After you reached your goal, it will be vital to maintain the new routines that you have created for yourself.

If you have been bringing healthy snacks to work, keep doing it. If you are exercising three days a week, keep doing it. If you are taking well-deserved breaks which help you work and worry less, keep doing this too. Keep up every positive habit you gained as you've implemented your plan.

Your energy level can decline quickly if you are not careful. Reaching your goal does not mean that you can let go of the things that got you here.

To keep your momentum going, do the following:

- Recall why you wanted high energy in your career and keep this thought alive daily.
- Continue to review your vision, plan, and calendar every day.
- Reward yourself for keeping your new routines in place.
- Remember to take one day at a time.

High energy will stay with you as long as you work to maintain it.

START YOUR NEXT PLAN

Now that you have your energy back, what's next?

Your career can span thirty, forty, fifty, or more years, so there will likely be time to do all of the things that you have always wanted to do. So, what do you want to do?

What do you see yourself doing in the future? Write down your thoughts, and start a new plan. Knowing that you have reached your high-energy goal can give you the confidence to take on just about any other goal you can think of.

Once you have regained your lost energy, you will feel that anything is possible. And you will be ready to take on the world.

The Expert Opinions

This next section contains the words of some amazing people.

They've helped me get my energy back. I thank each one of these experts for touching my life and for changing the way I look and feel. I admire their positive outlook and their commitment to health, energy, and vitality.

I asked each expert a series of questions about situations that are possibly draining your energy level at work. Most of the questions are the same; what is different is their answers.

Their wisdom is golden. Their words are priceless. I hope you benefit from their advice as much as I have.

KIMBERLY BREHM AND LINDA DUNLAP

Kimberly Brehm and Linda Dunlap
The Fitness Studio, 583 Montauk Highway, Eastport, NY 11941
631-325-2955
fitnessstudio@aol.com

Kimberly Brehm and Linda Dunlap are the owners of the Fitness Studio in Eastport, New York. Kimberly has a bachelor of science degree in kinesiology from the University of Maryland. Kimberly has been teaching aerobics for twelve years and has been a personal trainer for eight. Linda is a licensed physical therapy assistant. Linda has been teaching aerobics for twelve years and has been a personal trainer for ten.

Kimberly and Linda have created an amazing workout facility where you can work out and have a good time too. They are loving, accepting, and motivating people. I go to the Fitness Studio every morning. It is often the most enjoyable part of my day.

Kimberly and Linda, is it possible to have a high amount of energy at work?

You can have a high amount of energy at work, though it is important to remember that energy *balance* is the key. If you are fit, well rested, and well-balanced, you can have high levels of productivity.

What keeps people from feeling great at work every day?

There are numerous demands at work. Often, you have no control over these demands. Time constraints, external stresses, and deadlines—as well as strained relationships with co-workers—are some main causes of energy drain. Lack of control over these issues can lead to unhealthy choices if you are not careful.

If you are consistently tired at work, what is a healthy way to get more energy?

Movement is one of the most effective ways of increasing your energy. Movement does not have to be complex. Simple stretches at your desk will increase blood-flow. Here are some examples:

Spine-lengthening stretch—Stand next to a desk, put your hands on the surface, and bend forward from your waist (at a ninety-degree angle). Breathe in deep and pull your abdominals in as you exhale, lengthening from your tailbone to the top of your head. With each exhale, slide your hands forward to stretch more.

Hip flexor and calf stretch—Stand behind a chair and hold on lightly. Place one foot forward and one foot back, toes facing forward. Bend your front knee and straighten your back leg until your heel is on the floor. Press your hips forward and hold the position for twenty or thirty seconds. Then switch legs and repeat.

Lumbar release—Stand with feet hip-width apart and place your hands on your thighs above your knees. Bend your knees and lean forward from your waist so that your back is parallel with the floor. In this position, inhale through your nose and arch the back, dropping your belly button toward the floor. Then exhale and pull your abdominals in, rounding the back and dropping the chin toward the chest. Repeat.

You are at your desk and you have three large projects to finish by 5:00 PM. You are hungry. You look over and see that your co-worker has a large bowl of candy sitting on her desk. What do you do?

When faced with an immediate distraction, it is important to get control of your thought process. Start by closing your eyes and counting to ten slowly, aloud or in your head. Bring the focus back to the task you are trying to complete. If this doesn't work, stand up and walk over to the water cooler. Drink a glass of water. Water will fill your stomach and make you less likely to want to eat. If all else fails, ask your co-worker to remove the bowl of candy from her desk. If she refuses, ask if she could at least move it out of your field of vision—out of sight, out of mind.

It's your boss's birthday. The department chips in and gets him a cake. Everyone is eating a piece, including your boss and other people whom you would like to impress. The cake looks delicious. It's 3:00 PM, and you could use a boost to help you finish the day. What do you do?

First off, it's important to remember that it's OK to have a piece of cake once in a while. However, if this is what you choose as a source of energy on a regular basis, you'll have to remember that after you feel the boost, you will shortly feel the exact opposite, sluggish and tired. There are better sources of energy that will have a much longer lasting effect. Try to keep something around such as almonds or yogurt, so that you can participate in the snacking and not feel left out.

You have a big presentation to give tomorrow. All you can think about is doing a good job. It's 6:00 PM, and you are still at your desk. What can you do to make sure you are in the best possible mental and physical condition before tomorrow's presentation?

Make sure you get enough sleep. Get into bed early that night. If you are stressed or having difficulty sleeping, try running through your presentation to clear your head. Imagine that your presentation runs smoothly with no problems. This type of mental imagery can help your performance greatly. It is also important to have a healthy breakfast, such as oatmeal and fresh fruit. When your body is nourished, it is much easier to maintain concentration. Finally, be sure to be well hydrated.

You are tired. Your child was sick and kept you up all last night. You have a meeting with you boss in an hour. What can you do to get more energy for that meeting?

Physical activity releases endorphins that can help you be alert for the meeting. Do simple stretches. Stand up tall and reach your arms over your head. Inhale through your nose, and then exhale through your mouth as you open your arms wide. Bring your hands down by your hips and drop your chin to your chest. Do this three or four times, right before your meeting.

You want to go to night school in order to advance your career. But your day job is stressful and demanding. What can you do to get the energy to do both?

Balance is the key in this situation. Finding time to go to school while holding down a demanding career is challenging, so you need discipline and planning. To have a good amount of energy all day long, a well-balanced diet and daily exercise is imperative. Try starting your day with a twenty-minute yoga session (there are many great yoga DVDs you can buy on the market today), followed by a wholesome breakfast.

You want to start a healthy new phase in your life and career. What are some steps you can take? Where is the best place to start?

It is important to understand what being healthy encompasses. Health involves not only diet and exercise, but also rest, relaxation, and a well-rounded, enjoyable life. An easy way to start is to include physical activity. Start by walking for ten minutes every day, and slowly increase that amount to an hour. Another important aspect to tackle is nutrition. Take a look at your diet. It may help to consult a nutritionist to get you on the right path. Finally, look at your overall lifestyle. If your only outlet is work, it is important that you find other ways to balance this out. If you don't have any hobbies, try taking up something that isn't too time-consuming. There are a lot of options, but it is important to find one that makes your life more enjoyable. You may even find that walking becomes a hobby, and that you will begin to miss it if you cannot do it one day.

You have begun to eat better. You have even started an exercise program. Your boss walks in and tells you to pack your bags. You are going overseas. What can you do to make sure that you take your healthy new habits with you?

Write down what you are eating, when you are eating it, and what exercises you are doing. Bring what you wrote to your new location. This will be a very important reference to help you to stay on track.

What are some simple, practical, and easy-to-follow steps you can take to have more energy at work and feel great every day?

- Sleep—be sure to get to bed early on a consistent basis.
- Exercise—daily cardiovascular activity even in small amounts can help enormously.
- Eat well—eating less refined sugar and processed foods and more whole foods to boost overall energy levels.
- Set goals—it's much easier to stay motivated and energetic when you are working toward something specific.

What are some simple, practical, and easy-to-follow steps you can take to be healthier outside of work, which might help you to feel great and have more energy at your job every day?

A simple workout routine will help you stick to your goals. Start small and work up to more. Ten minutes will become twenty minutes and then thirty minutes relatively quickly with some consistency. Whatever steps you are taking, be sure to start slowly. If you try to force new habits all at once, you will find it much more difficult to sustain the changes.

What would you say to someone who says "I have no time" or "I have no energy" to implement the steps you've suggested?

There is hidden time in everyone's day; it just has to be located. For example, how long do you wait in line for coffee or breakfast in the morning? Maybe five minutes. Do you surf the Internet? Maybe thirty minutes. Do you take smoke breaks? Ten minutes. If you make some minor adjustments to the time you are spending on other things, that forty-five minutes is more than enough time to make changes. If you don't find the time for yourself, you will inevitably have to make the time later for illness and recovery.

If people had high energy, what would be possible for them in their careers?

The possibilities are limitless, depending of course on how focused you are and how much effort you are willing to put forth to making certain changes. Your energy levels correlate to your efforts and ultimately to your success.

What steps would you consider essential to a high-energy career success plan?

Writing down your plan and specifically defining the steps you need to take to reach your goals is extremely important. This will give you an action plan which you can reference often and keep you on track. Remember to be specific.

Is there anything else you would like to add?

It is important that you are realistic when you set goals for yourself. Goal setting can help you track your fitness *and* career progress. Setbacks will happen as well—this is something we all have to accept. They won't break you as long as you can get back on track quickly. Your career and your body are similar—the more effort you put forward, the more you will reap the benefits. The exciting part is that it gets easier over time.

BOB MITTLEMAN

Bob Mittleman, Owner, Fitness Together Personal Training Studio
8243 Jericho Turnpike, Woodbury, NY 11797
516-282-3000
www.ftwoodbury.com
bobmittleman@fitnesstogether.com

Bob is amazing. He currently owns and operates two Fitness Together personal training franchises in New York, with more on the way. Bob changed careers after spending eighteen years on Wall Street. He turned his passion for fitness into a career helping people improve their health and be in the best possible shape. Watching Bob progress in his career has been an inspiration to me.

Bob has completed eight marathons, finishing in the top 7 percent in each race. His personal best time is three hours and seven minutes. Aside from running marathons, he is active on the local running circuit and is the former coach of the Greater Long Island Running Club Racing Team. In addition to owning personal training studios, Bob also coaches people on how to run correctly. His clients range from the inexperienced to the advanced.

Bob, is it possible to have a high amount of energy at work?

Yes. It depends on attitude, focus, self-esteem, and what is being done by the individual to handle stress.

What keeps people from feeling great at work every day?

The day-to-day happenings can be a drag at times. This pertains to what goes on at the office and what is going on in the individual's personal life. It's ultra-important to have a clear head in order to get the most out of the day. A way to get a clear head is by keeping a journal. Keeping a journal is a great way to get what is in your head down on paper. It allows you see the way you are thinking. It allows you to strategize for the future as well as to look back. Too often, we get stuck in a rut and don't recognize our accomplishments either professionally or personally. Keeping a journal is a big help in alleviating this matter. Another way to feel great is to exercise. Exercise is a huge help in relieving stress and building awareness of one's body and surroundings.

If you are consistently tired at work, what is a healthy way to get more energy?

Take a short break. While doing so, perhaps go for a walk and get some water. The general formula is to drink the same number of ounces as half your weight in pounds. Ideally, one should drink anywhere from seventy-two to ninety-six ounces of water a day. This does not include coffee, tea, or soft drinks. In addition, walking is probably the best exercise option you will have available while at work. You can walk during your lunch break. Stretching is another good option. Stretching will help move your blood around, and you will feel better afterward. One stretch is the simple touch-your-toes stretch, without bending your knees. Do not bounce. Bend over and touch your toes and hold the position for a count of ten. Come up and do it again. Five repetitions should do the trick. Another good stretch is taking your arm and bringing it across your body. While doing so, take your free arm, wrap it around the arm across the body, and pull it toward you. Count to ten, and repeat five times for each arm. This can make a big difference.

You are at your desk and you have three large projects to finish by 5:00 PM. You are hungry. You look over and see that your co-worker has a large bowl of candy sitting on her desk. What do you do?

Do not take the candy. Candy does nothing to satisfy hunger. You may also feel guilty for eating the candy. Guilt will throw off your focus and prevent you from finishing your projects.

It's your boss's birthday. The department chips in and gets him a cake. Everyone is eating a piece, including your boss and some other people whom you would like to impress. The cake looks delicious. It's 3:00 PM, and you could use a boost to help you finish the day. What do you do?

You can have a small piece if you are eating for political reasons, but not for a boost to finish the day. Maybe you could have fruit or cold veggies instead. You could even get away with eating plain popcorn or pretzels. Make the choice that is right for you. You do not have to participate in every celebration.

You have a big presentation to give tomorrow. All you can think about is doing a good job. It's 6:00 PM, and you are still at your desk.

What can you do to make sure you are in the best possible mental and physical condition for tomorrow's presentation?

Relax and reread your presentation. Then do a practice run so that you are familiar and comfortable with the material. Practice one more time, and call it a day. Practice will give you the confidence to succeed. Get a good night's sleep. A good-paced walk would help as well. You can even practice your presentation while walking, if you want to.

You are tired. Your child was sick and kept you up all last night. You have a meeting with your boss in an hour. What can you do to get more energy for that meeting?

I think the best way to get more energy in this case is to have a good breakfast, to make sure you have consumed sixteen ounces of water or more, and to think positively about what needs to be accomplished at the meeting. A brief exercise routine such as fifty jumping-jacks, a hundred sit-ups, or forty or fifty push-ups can also add some needed energy.

You want to go to night school in order to advance your career. But your day job is stressful and demanding. What can you do to get the energy to do both?

You need to decide on a plan of action that will not drain your energy resources. It might make sense to write down the positives and negatives of attending night school. Once you have a better idea of what it will involve, you will feel better about attending. Drink lots of water. Stay away from caffeinated and sugary drinks. In the end, these will make you tired. Fitness can help. As you get more fit, your ability to endure harder and longer days will improve.

You want to start a healthy new phase in your life and career. What are some steps you can take? Where is the best place to begin?

It would make sense to begin with an exercise routine that incorporates weight training, cardio, and diet. The best place to start is with a personal trainer who can coach you as well as motivate you to reach your short and long-term goals. You might also want to seek the guidance of a nutritionist. Many people believe they *only* have to diet or *only* do cardio or *only* do weight training. This is not true. All three are needed in order to become energized.

You have begun to eat better. You have even started an exercise program. Your boss walks into your office and tells you to pack your bags. You are going overseas. What can you do to make sure that you take your healthy new habits with you?

You need to stay accountable to yourself. Map out your exercise routine prior to leaving. Find a hotel that has a workout facility. Log your activities while you are away. Your log should contain what exercises you are doing each day, what your intake of fluids are for each day, how much sleep you are getting, and what foods you are eating.

What are some simple, practical, and easy-to-follow steps you can take to have more energy at work and feel great every day?

- Drink more water throughout the day, anywhere from seventy-two to ninety-six ounces.

- Eat properly. You will know whether you are doing this or not. Questions to ask yourself are: Am I eating pasta every day? Am I eating cookies every day? Am I eating fried foods? Am I eating junk foods? Choose foods that are better for you.

- Exercise regularly—four to five times a week for thirty to sixty minutes.

- Keep a journal. Write down what you eat and drink and the exercises you have done. Also include your feelings for that day and your goals for the next day and beyond.

What would you say to someone who says "I have no time" or "I have no energy" to implement the steps you've suggested?

Those are excuses, and they make you weak. You need to *make* the time. See where your time is spent. Analyze your day. Analyze how important energy is to you. If it is important to you to find more energy and feel great, then you can find a way to fit in what I am suggesting.

If people had high energy, what would be possible for them in their careers?

Anything they want. It's not just the high energy, but also the focus that comes along with it. When you are focused and alert, you are more productive. You are also able to think more clearly and make better, stronger decisions about your job and career.

What steps would you consider essential to a high-energy career success plan?

Surround yourself with positive influences. Some may be external, and others may be internal. External sources can be friends, loved ones, coaches, and support groups. Internal influences come from you. You make yourself better by increasing your chances for success. Exercise regularly, eat well, and drink water consistently. It also helps to read motivational or self-help books.

Is there anything else you would like to add?

I have seen what stress can do to people. I have seen the ups and downs of many careers. I also speak freely about my own personal experiences. When I was working on Wall Street, as well as in my current position, I use exercise—for me, running—to keep me going throughout the day and the week ahead. Running has elevated my game to levels that few can comprehend. It has helped me stay focused and has given me the drive to succeed when otherwise I might have had none.

JEANETTE ZIRPOLI

Jeanette Zirpoli is a registered dietitian who is employed at a respected health-care facility on Long Island, NY. Jeanette has worked in various health care settings, from nursing homes, hospitals, and home-care to dialysis. She is a graduate of Queens College, CUNY, and is in the process of becoming a registered nurse, so that she can expand her horizons within the health care system. Jeanette is not accepting new clients at this time.

I have learned a lot from her about being healthy. Jeanette cares tremendously about diet and nutrition and is a wonderful role model for having a great career and a strong body. She is a passionate mother of two and is dedicated to teaching her children healthy habits at a young age. Jeanette is happily married to Darrin—an incredible person and great friend to my husband and me.

Jeanette, is it possible to have a high amount of energy at work?

Yes, if you can get adequate amounts of sleep every night, eat lean, well-balanced meals, and can incorporate daily physical activity into your routine.

What keeps people from feeling great at work every day?

Stress, tiredness, unhealthy eating, and lack of physical activity.

If you are consistently tired at work, what is a healthy way to get more energy?

Do not skip meals. Eating the right types of foods is important for energy. At your desk, keep healthy, low-fat snacks for quick pick-me-ups—a small bag of trail mix, or low-fat granola bars. Dried apricots, berries, or an apple would also be good choices. Fruit provides vitamins, minerals, fiber, and phytochemicals that increase the body's energy levels. If you have no option but to grab something from a vending machine, look for pretzels, because they will keep you feeling satisfied longer.

You are at your desk and you have three large projects to finish by 5:00 PM. You are hungry. You look over and see that your co-worker has a large bowl of candy sitting on her desk. What do you do?

Try to refrain from eating the candies; empty calories will do nothing more than provide a quick sugar rush that will leave you feeling hungry and cause you to crash later. Choose water instead, as sometimes thirst can be mistaken for hunger.

It's your boss's birthday. The department chips in and gets him a cake. Everyone is eating a piece, including your boss and some other people whom you would like to impress. The cake looks delicious. It's 3:00 PM, and you could use a boost to help you finish the day. What do you do?

You can allow yourself to splurge on a small piece, once in a while, on special occasions. But if you are an all-or-nothing person, high-sugar and high-fat foods will wear you out. If this is you, pass on the cake and choose a healthy snack instead.

You have a big presentation to give tomorrow. All you can think about is doing a good job. It's 6:00 PM, and you are still at your desk. What can you do to make sure you are in the best possible mental and physical condition for tomorrow's presentation?

If the work you're still doing at 6:00 PM is unrelated to the presentation the following day, call it a night, go home, and try to get as much rest as possible. It will help to have a clear head the next day. Try to avoid alcohol—even though it initially reduces tension and increases energy, it's a depressant and will cause an energy dip later on. The most important thing is to not skip breakfast the next morning. Do not eat a high-fat/high-calorie breakfast, such as eggs and sausage or pancakes with syrup, and avoid caffeine, which may perk you up temporarily but can cause restlessness and agitation once the jolt fades.

You are tired. Your child was sick and kept you up all last night. You have a meeting with your boss in an hour. What can you do to get more energy for that meeting?

That morning, during your shower, lather up with a citrus-scented soap—according to aromatherapy, the scent promotes alertness and relaxation. Then as you are getting dressed, try listening to your favorite type of music to lift your spirits. Make sure that your breakfast consists of a protein and a carbohydrate, because this will make your meal take longer to digest, thus helping keep your energy higher for a longer period of time. An example of such a breakfast would be a half cup of oatmeal and a hard-boiled egg, or nonfat yogurt with berries. In addition, organize and have everything ready that you will need for the meeting. If you are driving to work, park a distance from the office and walk briskly to help get your adrenaline pumping. If you work in a city and take public transportation, the hustle and bustle in the morning rush is adrenaline enough.

You want to go to night school in order to advance your career. But your day job is stressful and demanding. What can you do to get the energy to do both?

Take only one class at a time. Don't push yourself to do more than you might be able to handle. Most likely, it would be your school work that would suffer, and you wouldn't want to have to repeat the course if you fail.

You want to start a healthy new phase in your life and career. What are some steps you can take? Where is the best place to begin?

The best place to start is toward better health. First, eliminate unhealthy habits in your life. For example, if you're a couch potato, start by changing your behavior and routines. Instead of plopping down on the couch after eating, make it a point to take a daily fifteen-minute walk around the neighborhood, eventually picking up the pace and staying out longer. If you're a smoker or drinker, now is the time to quit. If you can make your life healthier, then you can have the right mind-set to focus on a career move or other change. For a healthy plan in your career, take a few moments to think about how you feel about your current job, and where you want to be in five years. What will it take to accomplish this? If you plan short-term goals to work toward, your career can change in a positive way.

You have begun to eat better. You have even started an exercise program. Your boss walks into your office and tells you to pack your bags. You are going overseas. What can you do to make sure that you take your healthy new habits with you?

There is certainly no excuse for not being able to continue your healthy new habits. Keep portions small and meals balanced whenever possible. Do not skip meals, and keep low-fat, healthy snacks such as fresh fruits or veggies on hand for those times when you find yourself hungry and wanting to munch on something. Remain physically active. You don't always have to go to a gym to exercise. Take the stairs instead of the elevator. Park your car a block away from your destination. Find the closest mall and walk a few brisk laps around it. If you have a choice of hotels, see whether any of them have a gym or swimming pool.

What are some simple, practical, and easy-to-follow steps you can take to have more energy at work and feel great every day?

Reduce your caffeine intake to one or two cups of caffeinated beverages a day, if you are someone who drinks a lot of caffeine. Caffeine can deter you from getting a sufficient amount of rest—you will find yourself needing more and more, and eventually you will crash. Do not consume too much soda, which is nothing more than sugar water. If you like juice drinks realize that these contain a lot of calories as well, so keep the serving-size to a maximum of six ounces daily.

Do not skip meals. Ideally, stick to three meals a day, with two or three healthy, low-fat snacks in-between to prevent yourself from feeling starved and ultimately making the wrong food choices. Avoid white flour and refined sugar. Try to keep your meals lean. Even though everyone needs a certain amount of fat in their diet, in our society most people well exceed this amount. Fats get stored on your hips, thighs, and abdomen and eventually can lead to health complications and depletion of your physical energy. Stay away from fried foods, foods accompanied by gravies or cream sauces, and breaded or battered foods. Steamed, boiled, or grilled foods are better choices than sautéed, because usually very little fat is used in these methods of cooking.

What are some simple, practical, and easy-to-follow steps you can take to be healthier outside of work, so that you can feel great and have more energy at your job every day?

Follow the same suggestions as in the last response, plus ensure that you get at least eight hours of sleep per night. If sleep is difficult for you, incorporating physical activity—no less than two hours before bedtime—may help to bring on sleepiness. If you're juggling a career with family, make time for yourself. It can be quiet time—relaxing in a bath using aromatherapy such as candles or scented oils in the bathwater, or curling up and reading a book. This will help reduce your stress levels considerably.

What would you say to someone who says "I have no time" or "I have no energy" to implement the steps you've suggested?

These statements are excuses. When it becomes important enough to you, you will find the time. Change does not have to happen all at once; take one step at a time, until the new behavior almost becomes second nature, and then move on to the next.

If people had high energy, what would be possible for them in their careers?

They may be able to think more clearly. They may be able to take on more tasks. They may become more productive. They may be able to do the extracurricular tasks needed in order to make a lateral move or a career change.

SUSAN 'SURYA' SEMERADE

Susan 'Surya' Semerade, RYT, CAP
PO Box 645, Speonk, NY 11972
516-381-3653
Livingayurveda@aol.com

Susan is an incredible healer who is dedicated to health, mind, body, and spirit. She is a Certified Ayurvedic Practitioner and a Certified Sivananda Yoga instructor. I take Susan's yoga classes on Sunday mornings. They are tough, but in a good way. I've learned that yoga is about letting go and being who you are and where you are in the moment. I am amazed that by allowing yoga into my life, I have gained strength and energy that I never thought possible. Susan has been a big part of my transformation and quest to make my dream of greater energy a reality.

Susan, is it possible to have a high amount of energy at work?

It is possible to maintain a high amount of energy at work, provided that you take care of yourself. With a healthy diet, a good night's sleep to restore and recharge the body, time made for hobbies and exercise, and some sort of meditation to relax and calm your delicate nervous system that has been on overdrive, you can sustain the energy that is required to keep up with the fast-paced and goal-oriented society that we live in.

What keeps people from feeling great at work every day?

Diet and how you eat your food are important factors to overall well-being. Your body will sooner or later begin to feel the effects of eating poorly. Excessive dining out or grabbing a quick snack from the fast food chains, combined with a lack of the energy needed to prepare wholesome meals, will take a toll on your body and energy level. In addition, eating quickly hampers your digestive process, which over time may lead to obesity, bloating, constipation, diarrhea, heartburn, headaches, insomnia, fatigue, and general malaise. What and how you eat can determine whether you feel great or not.

If you are consistently tired at work, what is a healthy way to get more energy?

A good way to restore energy is to take a short brisk walk in the sunshine to rejuvenate and recharge your batteries. When going out of doors is not an option, try some stretching or deep breathing, which can help reverse the tiredness. If possible, find a yoga studio in your area and sign up for a class. You will be amazed at what one hour per week at a yoga class can do for you.

You are at your desk and you have three large projects to finish by 5:00 PM. You are hungry. You look over and see that your co-worker has a large bowl of candy sitting on her desk. What do you do?

Who wouldn't love to dive into that bowl of candy? To help prevent you from plunging your hand in, you need to do some planning. Everyone needs a certain amount of "sweet" taste to maintain tissue development, but not the white refined sugars in candy—that has been stripped of any nutritional value. Keep a bag of unsalted nuts (preferably organic) in your desk drawer for just such an occasion. Nuts are high in protein and enhance memory and creativity. Mix up a batch of various nuts, add some raisins, and keep it in a container in your desk. The combination can help satisfy your sweet tooth. Just remember to chew the nuts slowly.

It's your boss's birthday. The department chips in and gets him a cake. Everyone is eating a piece, including your boss and some other people whom you would like to impress. The cake looks delicious. It's 3:00 PM, and you could use a boost to help you finish the day. What do you do?

There is nothing wrong with one piece of cake, once in a while. Most foods taken in moderation are OK. Keep in mind that sugar, like salt, is addicting; and if you're already hungry, you may feel compelled to go back for seconds. Remember to stock your desk drawer with healthy alternatives, like a nutritious energy bar or a container of dried fruit. If you munch on them during the day, you may be less likely to overindulge, and may be satisfied to eat a small sliver of cake to be polite.

You have a big presentation to give tomorrow. All you can think about is doing a good job. It's 6:00 PM, and you are still at your desk.

What can you do to make sure you are in the best possible mental and physical condition for tomorrow's presentation?

Have a restful night sleep so that you can be alert and functioning the next day. If sleep is difficult for you under normal circumstances, chances are it will be nearly impossible when your mind is in overdrive. To promote good sleep, take a nice warm bath with some calming lavender oil. In fact, put a few drops of this essential oil on your pillow just before going to bed. A glass of warm milk with a pinch of nutmeg has been known to induce sleep. Just before your presentation, take a few long, deep breaths—inhaling and exhaling through the nose until you feel calm and relaxed.

You are tired. Your child was sick and kept you up all last night. You have a meeting with your boss in an hour. What can you do to get more energy for that meeting?

Breathe properly. When you're tense and tired, you tend to take shallow breaths, only filling your upper lungs. This way of breathing is not enough to give you energy. Deep inhalations with long exhalations provide energy and improve mental concentration.

You want to go to night school in order to advance your career. But your day job is stressful and demanding. What can you do to get the energy to do both?

If your night classes begin directly after your work hours, plan ahead. On those evenings that you have school, eat a hearty lunch and then have some fruit before you leave the office. If possible, take a few minutes to breathe, with deep, long inhalations and exhalations. A proper amount of sleep the evenings before class nights will also have you feeling rejuvenated.

To help ease the stress in your workplace, set some boundaries and do your best to abide by them. Take your lunch hour—do not gulp down a container of yogurt at your desk with the phone at your ear and your fingers on the keyboard. Get up and away from your desk and preferably away from your office. Find a quiet place to eat wholesome food, and chew your food slowly and mindfully. Let co-workers know this is *your* time. This will give you energy for your nighttime studies.

You want to start a healthy new phase in your life and career. What are some steps you can take? Where is the best place to begin?

A good place to begin would be a visit to the local health-food store—almost every town and city has one. In all of the health-food stores I've ever been in, there are bulletin boards filled with flyers and business cards of professionals in various health fields. Contact one of them, so that you can set off on your path with an experienced person who can set you in the right direction.

Also, talk to one of the store employees—they are usually helpful and informative. They can suggest a book to get you started, or may even recommend a particular health professional you can call. The doors are wide open for you from there.

You have begun to eat better. You have even started an exercise program. Your boss walks into your office and tells you to pack your bags. You are going overseas. What can you do to make sure that you take your healthy new habits with you?

Regardless of your destination, or how long the flying time, traveling usually creates some challenges. Time changes, jet lag, lack of adequate sleep, airline food, and foods of different countries all cause havoc on your body. A first step would be to pack plenty of healthy snacks, a piece or two of fruit (orange, apple, or banana), and some herbal teabags in your carry-on, which you can have while in the air to avoid eating overcooked processed airline food. Be sure to drink plenty of bottled water and to stretch whenever you can, especially before and after a long flight. Once you have settled in and familiarized yourself with your new location (maybe there is a gym or yoga studio in the area—many hotels have one or both on the premises), make a reasonable schedule for yourself that is similar to the one you had at home. Do the best you can under the circumstances, and don't be too hard on yourself if you aren't able to follow through. Once you are back home, you can pick up where you left off.

What are some simple, practical, and easy-to-follow steps you can take to be healthier outside of work, so that you can feel great and have more energy at your job every day?

To maintain energy in the workplace, you need to live a healthy lifestyle. When you are burdened with worries and stress in other areas of your life, it will show up on the job. If you put all of your energy into your career, then your relationship or personal life may suffer as a consequence.

Following are some simple, practical, and easy steps to guide you toward feeling great.

- Begin with a visit to an Ayurvedic practitioner to help you determine your unique body constitution.
- Discover what foods are best for you and which ones to avoid.
- Create a simple yoga routine to do every morning before you start your day and one to do at the end of your day.
- Practice daily breathing techniques.
- Plan your day the night before, or even the week before. On days of long meetings or late hours, have meals prepared ahead of time.
- Keep healthy snacks and fruits handy at all times.
- Get adequate sleep.
- Make time for friends.
- Make time for family.
- Make time for yourself.
- Make time for quiet reflection.

Creating a healthy balance in all areas of your life takes thought and commitment. When you can accomplish that, you are healthy, you have energy, and you are happy. A visit to a good health professional can go a long way in helping you accomplish this goal.

What would you say to someone who says "I have no time" or "I have no energy" to implement the steps you've suggested?

The majority of us fall into the "every excuse in the book" category—I'll start my diet on Monday, when there's a new moon, when the kids go back to school, etc. The dedicated individual that makes a commitment to a healthy lifestyle is the exception to the rule.

Begin by making a plan and listing the things you want to achieve (as a high achiever you are probably already familiar with this method). Start with simple steps that can show quick results, such as finding a gym or yoga studio that fits into your schedule. Start with small changes in your diet—instead of three cups of coffee in the morning, have two. Replace sugar-coated cereal with a natural one free of additives.

Plan what you are going to wear the night before, to avoid that rushed feeling in the morning. Try going to sleep a half hour earlier and getting up a half hour earlier. This half hour will give you time for yourself. Recall the ancient Chinese proverb: "A journey of a thousand miles begins with a single step."

If people had high energy, what would be possible for them in their careers?

With high energy, anything is possible. The sky is the limit. But where is your energy coming from? Do you feel great naturally because you eat a well-balanced diet and a live a wholesome lifestyle? Or, is your high energy coming from sugar or caffeine? Balance is the key to a healthy and long life, which in turn, leads to possibilities in your career.

What steps would you consider essential to a high-energy career success plan?

All of what I have previously stated regarding diet and lifestyle would allow the energy required for a successful career. But I would have you question whether or not your career brings you happiness and have you ask yourself what happiness means to you. This is an important step in the process.

Is there anything else you would like to add?

As an Ayurvedic practitioner and a practicing yogini for over twenty-five years, I do my best to employ this ancient wisdom in the Western world and to encourage others to do so as well. At the birth of Ayurveda some four or five thousand years ago, the corporate world was unheard of.

Human beings have experienced stress since the days of fleeing from a predator. Although you no longer need to exhaust your energy fighting for your survival as your ancestors did, it's still important to come back to the basics—eating well, sleeping well, exercising, meditating daily, and creating time for your family, your friends, and yourself.

SARA GRAHAM ROYE

Sara Graham Roye
631-874-0070
www.saragraham.com

Sara is a certified Kripalu Yoga and meditation teacher. She graduated summa cum laude with a BA in philosophy, emphasizing world religion. Sara incorporates this knowledge into her teaching while guiding individuals to use their own intuitive knowledge to create meaningful yoga practices. Sara leads daily yoga classes and provides her students with individualized attention. She works with every student to adapt the practice to their own special needs and health issues.

What I love about Sara's yoga classes (I take them on Tuesday evenings) is that she brings both a calming sensibility and humor to her classes. Her style of teaching is fun-loving, spirited, and compassionate. We work hard, but I walk away feeling refreshed and energized. Sara believes that we should laugh and sweat every day. This is an inspiring principle to live by.

Sara, is it possible to have a high amount of energy at work?

Yes, it is possible as long as you keep a positive attitude and develop the willingness to commit to good health habits and routines.

What keeps people from feeling great at work every day?

Allowing outside influences and stress to weigh too heavily on them. Many people do not feel great at work because they don't invest the necessary amount of time into self-care. Spiritual depletion is another factor. Many people do not invest in their spiritual care.

If you are consistently tired at work, what is a healthy way to get more energy?

Learn yoga and Pranyama deep-breathing exercises to increase vitality and recharge your energetic batteries. Yoga teaches you how to develop a greater sense of connectedness and control of yourself, your body, and your energy. Pranayama teaches you how to move and control your energy. You can also get a nutritious recharge from a fresh raw juice drink or by eating whole, unrefined, unprocessed local foods.

You are at your desk and you have three large projects to finish by 5:00 PM. You are hungry. You look over and see that your co-worker has a large bowl of candy sitting on her desk. What do you do?

Everyone is different. Eating the candy may or may not affect how you feel. If you know yourself and believe that it will satisfy your appetite without destroying your energy once the sugar wears off, then eat it. The thing you want to avoid is eating the candy without even knowing that you're eating it. Try to notice when you act impulsively about food. Stop, take a deep breath, and listen. Ask yourself if you really want to eat this knowing how it will affect you, and act in a way that reflects your total needs. You may still want to eat that treat—and that's fine, as long as you are acting mindfully. It's all about making mindful choices. That alone will go a long way toward changing the way you feel.

It's your boss's birthday. The department chips in and gets him a cake. Everyone is eating a piece, including your boss and some other people whom you would like to impress. The cake looks delicious. It's 3:00 PM, and you could use a boost to help you finish the day. What do you do?

If you are well nourished, having a small slice of cake with everyone else should not do you any harm. If you want a treat every once in a while, make sure that you are eating plenty of good whole foods regularly, so that overall, you have optimum health and energy.

You have a big presentation to give tomorrow. All you can think about is doing a good job. It's 6:00 PM, and you are still at your desk. What can you do to make sure that you are in the best possible mental and physical condition for tomorrow's presentation?

Trust that you are ready. You have spent a lot of time with this material, so head home and focus on doing something relaxing that renews your sense of self as a human being, not a worker. Go to a yoga class, listen to a meditation CD, take a hot-tub bath, or go for a walk with a friend or family member. Have some tea and go to bed early, after setting out your clothes for tomorrow and arranging everything you will need to take with you to work. It is important that you make your presentation when you are at your best, so do what you need to do for self-care.

You are tired. Your child was sick and kept you up all last night. You have a meeting with your boss in an hour. What can you do to get more energy for that meeting?

Create a clear intention for the meeting, such as a desire to be open, relaxed, and helpful with your boss. Take some deep breaths and prepare for the meeting by taking a quick walk outside, or finding five minutes alone to do some deep breathing. It is possible that you're feeling exhausted because you need fresh air.

You want to go to night school in order to advance your career. But your day job is stressful and demanding. What can you do to get the energy to do both?

Treat your body as a temple. Simply being mindful about health and nutrition choices can make you feel like a whole new person—one who has the energy to undertake the challenge of additional schooling.

You want to start a healthy new phase in your life and career. What are some steps you can take? Where is the best place to begin?

Notice how your energy fluctuates throughout the day. Once you know when you naturally feel your best, you can try to schedule your appointments for these high-energy times of the day; and can schedule more mundane tasks for other times of the day.

You have begun to eat better. You have even started an exercise program. Your boss walks into your office and tells you to pack your bags. You are going overseas. What can you do to make sure that you take your healthy new habits with you?

Do your research. Know where you're going to be working out, eating, and shopping for good foods.

What are some simple, practical, and easy-to-follow steps you can take to be healthier outside of work, so that you can feel great and have more energy at your job every day?

Make your health a priority. Get good rest every day. Take time out to regroup. Eat healthy, varied meals. Consume a wide array of food types, including lean protein and simple local foods for maximum energy. Eliminate undue stress by organizing your home and workspace, so that you don't waste energy being rushed because you can't find your keys or anything to wear. Simplify. Don't waste energy on those activities that distract you from what is really important to you. Drink water.

Both at home and at work, create an environment that fosters feelings of peacefulness, so that you will feel more inspired and work more efficiently. Make rest a priority, as well as good nutrition—even if that means you have meals delivered to your home. Keep perspective on relationships, and do not let other people's problems and issues become your own. Try to not overextend yourself. Develop conscious boundaries. Living simply will preserve energy. Make an effort to stay in harmony with nature. Take care of yourself first, and all else will follow with more ease. Develop an awareness of gratitude. Ask for help when you need it. Set aside time and a place for exercising your breath and body. Fitness includes mind and body healing and maintenance.

What would you say to someone who says "I have no time" or "I have no energy" to implement the steps you've suggested?

No one can convince you that you must be healthier. But the truth is that once you begin, the results will motivate you to continue. The time and the energy that it takes to follow these steps will pay off so highly that you soon won't be able to imagine *not* following them.

If people had high energy, what would be possible for them in their career?

High energy and an honest life.

What steps would you consider essential to a high-energy career success plan?

Self care, consistency, finding a mentor, and helping others. Adding some sort of regular yoga, meditation, reiki, karate, or tai chi practice into your life will help as well. Select something that is your own, that will develop your spiritual and physical consciousness, and that will keep you grounded. In addition, prioritize your schedule to best utilize your natural energy levels and make the most of your body's rhythm.

Is there anything else you would like to add?

It is necessary to develop a consciousness of your energy tendencies before you can make real changes. Bramacharya (energy management) is a key principle in yoga which guides you to understand that using your energy properly, with the right people, will not exhaust or waste it. Wasteful relationships are ones that deplete you and prevent you from feeling alive and fulfilled.

JULIE A. VAN NOSTRAND

Julie A. Van Nostrand
21 Kettle Hole Road, Manorville, NY 11949
631-874-0104
Julesv34@aol.com

Julie holds a masters degree in school counseling and is currently pursuing an advanced professional diploma in marriage and family therapy. Julie was a senior editor at a pharmaceutical journal called *U.S. Pharmacist* and has assisted in the editing of two books: *School Counseling Principles Ethics and Law* and *The Transformed School Counselor,* the latter in which she was quoted. Julie has studied voice for over twenty-five years, and has been a soloist at various churches for more than twenty years. She has also performed at Carnegie Hall.

Julie and I work out together at the Fitness Studio, having interesting conversations while on our elliptical machines. Julie has various interests and is very passionately committed to them all. Julie is brilliant. She is the type of person that you stop and listen to when she speaks, because you know that she has something important to say.

Julie, is it possible to have a high amount of energy at work?

It is possible to have a high amount of energy at work. The key to having a high amount of energy is finding out what energizes you (and it does not have to be at work) and making it part of your life. It could be a daily thing like exercising, or taking tango lessons on the weekends. What recharges your battery will give you more energy at work and leave you with the feeling that there is more to your life than just your job.

What keeps people from feeling great at work every day?

People are people. By that I mean that the human condition is such that we are affected on a daily basis by a variety of factors. The weather, the stock market, spouses, and children can all keep people from feeling great at work, and that's OK. It's important to feel your feelings, whatever they are. But when you are not feeling great most of the time, it might be a good opportunity to look inside to see what is holding you back.

Many people change the scenery in their lives, but don't look carefully at what they bring to the workplace that might be an obstacle. If you've got appendicitis, a trip to Hawaii won't cure you; it will just change the place where you have appendicitis. An honest look at yourself may be just the thing to discover what is keeping you from feeling great at work and throughout life.

If you are consistently tired at work, what is a healthy way to get more energy?

Take a mental vacation and connect to the thing that personally energizes you. If you are charged up by thinking about a weekend on the beach, think about it. Close your eyes and think about the warm sand and lapping water. Picture yourself there. Allow yourself five minutes for a mental vacation.

You are at your desk and you have three large projects to finish by 5:00 PM. You are hungry. You look over and see that your co-worker has a large bowl of candy sitting on her desk. What do you do?

Louis Pasteur said, "Chance favors the prepared mind." So make a plan. Plan something healthy to eat and prioritize the projects that you must complete for the day. By having a plan in place, you can worry less about the deadline and concentrate more on your work. Don't let the saboteur at the next desk derail you from your true goals. By choosing to avoid the candy sitting on your co-worker's desk, you are making a good decision for your health and well-being, and you give your self-esteem a solid boost too.

It's your boss's birthday. The department chips in and gets him a cake. Everyone is eating a piece, including your boss and some other people whom you would like to impress. The cake looks delicious. It's 3:00 PM, and you could use a boost to help you finish the day. What do you do?

Have a piece of cake. The key to feeling great at work is being real. It's a birthday celebration, and celebrations often revolve around food. That's real. If there are people around whom you want to impress, be real with them, and have a bite or two of the cake. And starting a conversation with your boss by saying, "This cake is delicious" is not a bad opening. Workers who are honest, flexible, and real go far.

As for getting a 3:00 PM boost, it's really a decision you have to make. Will you feel worse about yourself afterward? Be true to yourself first. If that piece of cake will start you on a downward spiral of binge-eating and otherwise feeling bad about yourself, skip it. Talk to your boss about another subject that you think will work, and know that bosses and others are more interested in what you think and how you work than what you eat.

You have a big presentation to give tomorrow. All you can think about is doing a good job. It's 6:00 PM, and you are still at your desk. What can you do to make sure that you are in the best possible mental and physical condition for tomorrow's presentation?

Nobody knows you better than you. Some people operate fabulously on four hours of sleep. Others need eight or nine hours to feel refreshed and ready for the day. What is your style? Get the sleep *you* need. Some people like a hearty breakfast, while others feel sluggish after a full meal in the morning. Go with what you prefer.

Mentally, the best way to prepare for your presentation is to avoid getting caught up in what other people might be thinking about you and your work. Negative self-talk can make people so concerned about second-guessing their listeners' thoughts that their presentations lack the polish and drive that they need to be successful. So there you are, worried that your boss is not pleased with your work and the HR person is writing an ad for your job to appear in next week's paper. You have lost your focus, and your performance in delivering the material is nose-diving. You might know your material inside out, but right now your thoughts are elsewhere. Concentrate on the best job you can do and allow others their thoughts and feelings. When you are focused on your material, negative thoughts cannot creep in.

You are tired. Your child was sick and kept you up all last night. You have a meeting with your boss in an hour. What can you do to get more energy for that meeting?

If you were up all night with your sick child, there is no doubt that your thinking might be cloudy as you enter the meeting with your boss. Do the best you can. If you think it is appropriate, you can mention that you might not be as sparkling as usual because of the circumstances. If the climate at your job is not conducive to that kind of disclosure, don't mention it, but know inside that you are doing the best you can at balancing work and family. Cut yourself some slack. You'll be a better worker and parent.

You want to go to night school in order to advance your career. But your day job is stressful and demanding. What can you do to get the energy to do both?

Here, again, a plan is the way to go. Do you know what you want to study? Do you have a clear idea of how additional education will help you to advance in your career? Will an advanced degree or additional training reduce the stress or demands of your current job? Will the schooling you are contemplating be really tough on you and your schedule for a time, but set you up to be in a much better place in the long run? Are you energized by that idea? Suffering through graduate school or other kinds of training with no clear focus or direction can make the additional demands on your time unbearable. But with a plan and a clear beginning, middle, and end, the energy to get through will sustain itself.

You want to start a healthy new phase in your life and career. What are some steps you can take? Where is the best place to begin?

Begin by defining what healthy changes you would like to make. *Act as a consultant to yourself.* If you were called in to make some lifestyle changes on you, where would you likely begin? You may decide to stop smoking or take the stairs instead of the elevator. Build on small successes. If you skipped the greasy fries at lunch today in favor of some fresh fruit, you have begun. If you counted to ten before reacting to your co-workers in anger, you have already begun. Take notice of the small victories and watch your confidence grow. Perhaps the small changes you have made are the foundation for some really big changes ahead. *As the consultant*, you know the road that leads to success. Follow your designated path.

You have begun to eat better. You have even started an exercise program. Your boss walks into your office and tells you to pack your bags. You are going overseas. What can you do to make sure that you take your healthy new habits with you?

The key to success is that *you* have changed. Yes, you have created the environment that made the change possible, but you have changed your priorities and are making better decisions for your health and well-being. An unexpected business trip is not the time to abandon those good changes. Just as you created the environment that led to the current change, you must adjust the environment to keep the change relevant. The truth is that *you* are the only constant in the whole equation, and changes like an unexpected trip are going to come up. Plan for them. If you view yourself as the constant and can develop a plan based on flexibility, you are more likely to keep your healthy habits going, even if they aren't perfect all the time.

What are some simple, practical, and easy-to-follow steps you can take to have more energy at work and feel great every day?

Many people give all they have to their jobs and their families, which leaves little left for themselves. This is especially true for women who routinely juggle career and family and often find themselves worrying that they are not giving enough to either.

What if the recipe for feeling great at work is doing something positive for yourself every day, whatever that happens to be? What would those simple, practical, and easy-to-follow steps for feeling great at work look like for you? Don't worry that they are not readily accessible at all times. Take time to enjoy the journey of self-exploration that you have embarked on, and make the changes that feel most important to you.

What are some simple, practical, and easy-to-follow steps you can take to be healthier outside of work so that you can feel great and have more energy at your job every day?

Become comfortable with being uncomfortable. Let's say, for example, that you have been a smoker for your entire life. A persistent cough has brought you to the doctor's office (the cough made you uncomfortable). The doctor has some grim news. Without immediate changes in your habits you are facing long-term and near-certain terminal illness. The doctor's delivery is straightforward and serious. He needs to make sure you understand the gravity of your condition.

Now let's say that your medical prognosis has not changed, but your doctor has sweetened the delivery dramatically. If it's not too much trouble, you might try throwing the cigarettes away and lose some weight. But there is no need to hurry about it. Take your time. Feel comfortable. He does not want to make you unhappy, or force you to look at things that might disturb your rosy view of life. He wants to be a nice guy. Which doctor would you rather have take care of you? Discomfort is an invitation to change. Don't ignore it.

What would you say to someone who says "I have no time" or "I have no energy" to implement the steps you've suggested?

I would say that the person who says "I have no time" or "I have no energy" is really saying "I don't want to," or "I'm afraid"—and that's OK. At the end of the day, we are all driven by what we want and what we don't want. It might not be the best time for you to start if you have defeated yourself before you begin. Decide what you want, and then do it. That's the only way energy will happen for you.

If people had high energy, what would be possible for them in their careers?

Anything they wanted. People living with high energy tend to accomplish much more than people who do not.

Is there anything else you would like to add?

The answers in this section were written for the general population. If you find that you are struggling in life with a number of different things, professional help may be the answer. If you are depressed or addicted to something, please do not hesitate to contact your physician and get the help you need, so that you can more fully implement the suggestions contained in this section.

JOHN F. WHITAKER

John F, Whitaker, DC, LAc.
Whitaker Chiropractic
247 Main Street, Center Moriches, NY 11934
631-878-6262

John is a doctor of chiropractic and a licensed acupuncturist. He is dedicated to his profession and to learning something new each day. He is friendly, upbeat, and a terrific healer. If I have a pain in my back or a bloated stomach, I go to John's office, and I walk out feeling like a different person. John's partner is Jane Whitaker, his sister, who is also a chiropractor. Her knowledge of the body and her care in treating her patients is amazing. Together, they have helped me feel and look better. I am grateful to them both.

John, is it possible to have a high amount of energy at work?

Of course. Energy, like many other things, runs in cycles. It is always changing, both physically and mentally.

What keeps people from feeling great at work every day?

The problem (and the solution) is that we bring ourselves and our thoughts (both negative and positive) to work. On top of that, we are inundated by co-workers, bosses, customers, calls from family, etc. If you are well-balanced, you are better able to deal with the different forces that come at you.

If you are consistently tired at work, what is a healthy way to get more energy?

You could take a walk, take a few deep breaths, or put cold water on your face. This will help get your energy level up.

You are at your desk and you have three large projects to finish by 5:00 PM. You are hungry. You look over and see that your co-worker has a large bowl of candy sitting on her desk. What do you do?

Stay away from the candy. The long-term effect on the pancreas is not worth the quick energy fix. Also, relying on candy for energy can become a bad habit, affecting you negatively over the long haul.

It's your boss's birthday. The department chips in and gets him a cake. Everyone is eating a piece, including your boss and some other people whom you would like to impress. The cake looks delicious. It's 3:00 PM, and you could use a boost to help you finish the day. What do you do?

Eat a small piece. Tell your boss that you appreciate him/her and are enjoying the cake.

You have begun to eat better. You have even started an exercise program. Your boss walks into your office and tells you to pack your bags. You are going overseas. What can you do to make sure that you take your healthy new habits with you?

Make sure you get at least five servings of fruit and vegetables a day. In addition, stay away from refined carbohydrates, because they will slow you down.

What are some simple, practical, and easy-to-follow steps you can take to be healthier outside of work, so that you can feel great and have more energy at your job every day?

- Exercise daily.
- Eat well-balanced meals.
- Say positive affirmations each day.

What would you say to someone who says "I have no time" or "I have no energy" to implement the steps you've suggested?

Take one step at a time, day by day. If you slip up, start again.

If people had high energy, what would be possible for them in their careers?

Persistence. When obstacles arise, high energy keeps persistence alive.

What steps would you consider essential to a high-energy career success plan?

Select a worthy goal and judiciously analyze the necessary actions to reach it. Weigh the costs and benefits of reaching your goal, and then get started.

Is there anything else you would like to add?

Get to the root of why your energy is low. Modern medicine may give you systematic relief, but the underlying cause of your low energy may still go undetected.

JUDITH ROSE

Judith A. Rose, RN, LCSW, CHT
jrose@hypnosisbyjrose.com
www.hypnosisbyjrose.com
631-653-8664

Judith is a certified hypnotherapist, a licensed clinical social worker, and a registered nurse with more than twenty years of experience in the health care field. She is a member of the American Society of Clinical Hypnosis, as well as a member of numerous business and women's professional organizations.

Judith has worked with hundreds of people—helping them quit smoking, lose weight, and handle difficult personal and professional problems. Judith has developed a series of incredible audio programs (CDs and tapes) that either enhance the hypnotherapy experience for her clients, or help those who want to work on their own.

Judith is caring, enthusiastic, and great at what she does. Judith's biggest contribution to my energy level was regarding food. When I was working constantly, I depended on the wrong foods to give me energy. I gained weight and needed help with creating new eating habits. Judith helped me come to terms with why I was eating and introduced different techniques to prevent me from reaching for food when stressed. I got control of my eating, lost some weight, and I feel so much better.

Judith, is it possible to have a high amount of energy at work?

Yes, but it takes some planning and a good attitude.

What keeps people from feeling great at work every day?

A lot is about attitude—attitude about life, yourself, your job, and your physical and mental health. Also, you need to ask yourself how you feel about things. Do you like your job, or do you view it as drudgery? Are you overworked, underpaid, unappreciated, or not respected in the workplace? Do you feel stressed? What is your home life like? What kind of support do you have? Do you get enough sleep? What is most important is your perception. Do you feel like you are in control of your environment, or is your environment controlling you?

Perception, attitude, and gratitude are crucial in being energetic and feeling great at work or any other place. The good news is that you can change and improve your environment so that you can have a better quality of life.

You are consistently tired at work. What is a healthy way to get more energy?

Take five minutes to relieve stress. I have a stress-busting technique that I use with my clients. This technique can help reduce stress and increase energy. You can also use it to assist with visualizing your career goals. Here's what you do:

- Sit in a comfortable position.

- Pick a spot to stare at, straight ahead.

- While staring at the spot, start your "special" breathing. Special breathing consists of inhaling through your nose, slowly filling up your lungs, and then gently exhaling through your mouth, until you cannot comfortably breathe out any more. This should be a 1:2 ratio. That is, it should take you twice as long to exhale as to inhale.

- Take five slow and easy special breaths while staring at your spot.

- Now close your eyes and begin to imagine yourself in a beautiful place or achieving a specific goal.

- Make the visualization as real and compelling as you can—see what you would see, hear what you would hear, and feel what you would feel. If there are smells and tastes involved, include them too. The point is to make believe you are really there. For example, if your special place were a beach, what would you see there? Water, sand, boats, shells, etc. What would you hear there? The waves on the shore, birds, kids playing, etc. What would you feel there? The warmth of the sun, the touch of the sand, water, etc. Can you smell the salt air, or perhaps smell sun tan lotion? The point is to make it so real that it feels like you are really there.

- After two or three minutes, the picture or idea (as some people are not very visual) may fade away and that's OK.

- Allow your eyes to open, and enjoy a calmer, more relaxed you. For the first few minutes after opening your eyes and orienting yourself back in the room, you will usually feel very relaxed. Then usually ten minutes or so later, you will become more energized.

If you have any difficulty with this technique, please feel free to call me, and I will answer any questions that you may have.

You are at your desk and you have three large projects to finish by 5:00 PM. You are hungry. You look over and see that your co-worker has a large bowl of candy sitting on her desk. What do you do?

Get up, move around, and get something to drink instead, because often when you think you are hungry, you are actually thirsty. If you don't have a weight issue, a little of the candy won't hurt you, but after the initial energy boost, it may make you more tired than before.

It's your boss's birthday. The department chips in and gets him a cake. Everyone is eating a piece, including your boss and some other people whom you would like to impress in the company. The cake looks delicious. It's 3:00 PM, and you could use a boost to help you finish the day. What do you do?

As long as you are not diabetic, graciously take the cake. If you have weight issues, eat three to five bites. No one really cares if you eat the whole thing, and this way, you are a part of celebrating your boss too.

You have a big presentation to give tomorrow. All you can think about is doing a good job. It's 6:00 PM, and you are still at your desk. What can you do to make sure that you are in the best possible mental and physical condition for tomorrow's presentation?

Practice the five-minute stress-busting technique I described earlier, and visualize the presentation going exactly the way you want it to go. Do the stress-busting technique once before going to bed and again in the morning. Between tonight and tomorrow, give yourself a lot of positive self-talk and encouragement. The more you keep telling yourself that you are going to do well, the better your chances that you will. "What we believe about our selves becomes the truth for us," to quote Louise Hay.

You are tired. Your child was sick and kept you up all last night. You have a meeting with your boss in an hour. What can you do to get more energy for that meeting?

I can best answer this question by telling a story. One day years ago, I had difficulty sleeping. On this particular day, after getting only one hour of sleep, I woke up in tears knowing I had a very long and busy day ahead of me. I sat on the side of my bed and said to myself, "OK, Judith, this is your chance to practice what you tell others." I started to say out loud to myself, "I feel so good, I feel so good," over and over—sort of saying it, sort of singing it, louder and louder, as I walked to the shower. I passed the mirror and saw myself saying, "I feel so good," when, at that point, I really didn't. I started laughing about how silly it all seemed, but I kept it going. By the time I finished the shower, I was alert and energized. I couldn't believe how much better I felt. I got through the day and even had someone tell me I looked good. This was more proof to me that positive self-talk works. Positive affirmations and positive self-talk is imperative to feeling great.

You want to go to night school in order to advance your career. But your day job is stressful and demanding. What can you do to get the energy to do both?

I would want you to think about what taking on this extra commitment would really mean for you. Would it advance your career in a way that is truly your heart's desire? Or are you doing it for some other reason? Do you believe it is possible to have a job that you truly love, or do you see work as something that you have to grin and bear? Or something that you have little choice about?

Many people have a bad attitude about work because they do not like what they do, and they feel stuck. Their minds make them prisoners to jobs they do not enjoy. It would be hard to have high energy if this was your mind-set. Do some self-reflection. When you get quiet with yourself and listen to your intuition, you will find the answers, energy, and direction for your career.

You want to start a healthy new phase in your life and career. What are some steps you can take? Where is the best place to begin?

Take a personal inventory of your life and career. What is working, and what is not? What makes you happy, what gives you joy, and what does not? What is your physical health like? Are you overweight? Do you smoke? Do you have poor sleep habits? Do you exercise? What about the spiritual aspect of your life? What about gratitude? How do you see the proverbial glass of water—is it half full or half empty? Write your answers down so you have a place to begin. It is also important to repeat positive affirmations and listen to motivational tapes. Your goal is to stop the negativity. Get help to stop if you need it.

I personally feel that hypnotherapy is a great place to begin. There are so many benefits from hypnosis. It is great for relieving stress, for stopping smoking, and for losing weight. Treatment time is usually much shorter than traditional psychotherapy and could be both better for the busy person and easier on the pocketbook.

What would you say to someone who says "I have no time" or "I have no energy" to implement the steps you've suggested?

I hear this lot. I would say that they have come to me or are reading this book for a reason. Something in their life or career is not working the way they would like it to. They are unhappy, tired, or stressed out. I would ask them to think about this statement: "If you always do what you have always done, you will always get what you have always gotten." It is time to try something different. If they cannot take five or ten minutes a day to try something different, then it's time to ask for help, because their life is out of balance.

Is there anything you would like to add?

Most people are overworked, tired, stressed, overweight, unhealthy, and not finding much joy in their lives. This is because they are trying to do too much at once. Yes, I do believe that we can have it all, but without paying too steep a price. I do think that it is true when they say, "No one was ever lying on their deathbed wishing they had spent more time at work."

Be with the kids and enjoy them, or with your spouse, or traveling the world, or playing the violin. Remember, a joyful career is about balance. The better care you take now of your physical, mental, and spiritual health, the better your life and career will be. Remember also that we live in a medical age that will keep us alive for a long time. But what will our quality of life be like? How much pleasure will we have if we do not feel well? Much of how we feel when we get older is a direct result of the care we take of ourselves right now. Treat your body like the gift it is.

DEBORAH NEUBERGER

Deborah Neuberger
The Fitness Studio, 583 Montauk Highway, Eastport, NY 11941
631-325-2955
fitnessstudio@aol.com

Deborah Neuberger works at the Fitness Studio in Eastport, NY. She is Pilates-Certified, Physical Mind Institute Certified, an AFAA group fitness instructor, an AFAA personal trainer, and a business management graduate from Pace University.

Deborah is a great instructor. She believes that you should go at your own pace and listen to your body when you work out. I enjoy Deborah's Pilates classes very much, and am stronger and leaner because of them.

Deborah, is it possible to have a high amount of energy at work?

Yes, if you love what you do and enjoy the people you work with.

What keeps people from feeling great at work every day?

Stress and being in the wrong job.

If you are consistently tired at work, what is a healthy way to get more energy?

Fuel your body with good cuisine such as whole unprocessed foods, fruits, vegetables, and nuts. In addition, get up from your desk once in a while, and take a break.

You are at your desk and you have three large projects to finish by 5:00 PM. You are hungry. You look over and see that your co-worker has a large bowl of candy sitting on her desk. What do you do?

Concentrate on your work. Make a plan how you are going to get these projects done in the time you have, and assign time limits for each item. This will help you stay on track and focused. In addition, breathe. Most people are not aware that their breath becomes shallower and less effective as they get stressed. Breathing gives you energy and rejuvenation.

It's your boss's birthday. The department chips in and gets him a cake. Everyone is eating a piece, including your boss and some other people whom you would like to impress. The cake looks delicious. It's 3:00 PM, and you could use a boost to help you finish the day. What do you do?

Take a small piece of cake, walk around, and talk to the people. Be engaged in your conversations so that you are too occupied to eat the cake. If cake is one of your favorite foods, you can have a bite. Deprivation is not the answer. Decide beforehand how much you will eat, and then stick to your decision.

You have a big presentation to give tomorrow. All you can think about is doing a good job. It's 6:00 PM, and you are still at your desk. What can you do to make sure that you are in the best possible mental and physical condition for tomorrow's presentation?

Eat a healthy dinner that includes foods that are not overly processed. Good choices are vegetables and protein. This meal will fuel your body and brain. Avoid alcohol, because it will make you feel sluggish the next day. Get a good night's rest. Have a healthy breakfast the next morning. Before your presentation, stretch. Stretch your fingers to the ceiling. Shrug your shoulders a few times. Stretching will relax you and get you ready to do a good job.

You want to go to night school in order to advance your career. But your day job is stressful and demanding. What can you do to get the energy to do both?

Schedule everything. Put into your schedule moments for you, and try not to over-commit and add too many items to your plate. This will reduce your stress and increase the control and energy you have concerning your growing to-do list. When you get home, find some quiet time. Read, take a bath, or take a walk. This will help you stay in a healthy state of mind.

You have begun to eat better. You have even started an exercise program. Your boss walks into your office and tells you to pack your bags. You are going overseas. What can you do to make sure that you take your healthy new habits with you?

Work out, even if you have to exercise in your hotel room. Push-ups, crunches, and leg-lifts can make a difference. Plus, the movement will give you energy.

Keep up your good eating habits, eating foods that are processed as little as possible.

What would you say to someone who says "I have no time" or "I have no energy" to implement the steps you've suggested?

You just have to start. Making a commitment is always the hardest part. Once you commit, implementing the steps becomes easier. If you don't want to start alone, find a buddy to support and join you.

If people had high energy, what would be possible for them in their careers?

The sky's the limit.

Is there anything else you would like to add?

It's all about taking baby steps—one step at a time.

DOROTHY A. MORGAN

Dorothy A. Morgan, NPP, CHT
201 Montauk Highway, Suite 2, Westhampton Beach, NY 11978
631-831-4030

Dorothy Morgan is a board-certified psychiatric nurse practitioner and a certified hypnotherapist. She received a BSN from Columbia University's School of Nursing, an MSN from Stony Brook University, and a hypnotherapist certification from the National Guild of Hypnotists.

I work out with Dorothy at the Fitness Studio and we have a good time together at the gym. Dorothy is dedicated to her health and vitality, and I admire her commitment greatly. Dorothy loves what she does for a living, and I know that the devotion she has at the gym carries over to her clients.

Dorothy, is it possible to have a high amount of energy at work?

Yes. It is possible to be energized at work.

What keeps people from feeling great at work every day?

Not liking your job, being in the wrong type of work, not having a sense of purpose, or being out of balance.

If you are consistently tired at work, what is a healthy way to get more energy?

Take a small break of approximately ten or fifteen minutes, so you can get away from your work. You can take a short walk or close the door and meditate for several minutes. The goal is to clear your mind. In addition, get out at lunchtime. You will feel much more refreshed if you do.

It's your boss's birthday. The department chips in and gets him a cake. Everyone is eating a piece, including your boss and some other people whom you would like to impress. The cake looks delicious. It's

3:00 PM, and you could use a boost to help you finish the day. What do you do?

Ask yourself whether you really want the cake, or do you just want to fit in. If you just want to fit in, you can do so in other ways—through socializing and being interested in the other people in the room. Take the focus off yourself and focus on why you are there: a special occasion and an opportunity to celebrate your boss's birthday.

You have a big presentation to give tomorrow. All you can think about is doing a good job. It's 6:00 PM, and you are still at your desk. What can you do to make sure that you are in the best possible mental and physical condition for tomorrow's presentation?

Go home. Review your presentation. Then take a warm shower to calm your mind. Get a good night's sleep without medication—medication may make you feel groggy in the morning. If necessary, try a natural product such as Bach's Rescue Remedy to help you sleep. Never use alcohol to induce sleep. In the morning, review your presentation material again. If you are experiencing mild anxiety, accept it, since mild anxiety can be a motivating factor.

You want to go to night school in order to advance your career. But your day job is stressful and demanding. What can you do to get the energy to do both?

Most colleges now have weekend classes, which may accommodate your schedule in a more convenient manner. Most major colleges also have classes that can be taken online, so that you can do the work at any time of the day or night. Start by taking one class and work up from there. Use your commuting time, if you can, to do research or homework. Use your free time as efficiently as possible, and you'll feel better about both work and school.

You have begun to eat better. You have even started an exercise program. Your boss walks into your office and tells you to pack your bags. You are going overseas. What can you do to make sure that you take your healthy new habits with you?

This does not have to be an issue at all. People in most countries outside the United States do not consume the amount of junk food we do, or serve large portions the way this country does. Sticking to your new-found eating plan can be applied all over the world. Modify your exercise program by going out for walks, or taking your yoga mat with you and doing yoga in your hotel room. Inquire if the hotel you are staying at has bike rentals. Swim in the pool, if one is available. Most major hotels have some form of fitness center available. Modify, don't abandon, your eating and exercise program while away on business. If you stay open-minded and flexible, you may pick up on some new food ideas or exercise programs to take back with you.

What are some simple, practical, and easy-to-follow steps you can take to be healthier outside of work so that you can feel great and have more energy at your job every day?

Daily exercise is a positive stress-reducer and brings fresh oxygen to the brain. Getting quality sleep is much more important than how much sleep you get. If you do not go through the entire sleep cycle and are lacking in restorative sleep, then no amount of sleep is beneficial for you. Keep alcohol consumption to a reasonable level, since it does interfere with sleep and cognitive functioning. Don't isolate yourself. Studies have shown that socialization and laughter will make you feel better.

What would you say to someone who says "I have no time" or "I have no energy" to implement the steps you've suggested?

Claiming to have no time or energy means that change is not important enough to you. Prioritizing, goal-setting, effective scheduling, and developing achievable time frames are all imperative to obtaining anything that you want.

If people had high energy, what would be possible for them in their careers?

The question to ask yourself is, "If I were adequately energized, what would be possible in my life?" Success depends on being motivated, setting goals, and realistically working toward them. Success depends on overcoming situations which do not prove to be fruitful and knowing when to modify the overall direction of your life. Success depends on knowing that you do not know everything, and that in order to achieve success, you need the cooperation and support of others. Success requires a realistic time frame for attainment. Rarely is success achieved overnight.

What steps would you consider essential to a high-energy career success plan?

In order to achieve and enjoy success, you need to be balanced. If you are not, burnout will occur. If you want to stay ahead of the game and continue to be motivated, balance out your work life with your personal life. Be realistic with your goals. Know your limitations and work within them. Know when to modify a plan, or when to scrap it.

In addition, include vacations in your plan. Research suggests that individuals who take at least one vacation a year live approximately six years longer. A vacation means getting away from your usual routine and environment. Taking your computer and answering work-related calls while away does not constitute a vacation. Similarly, staying home for a week or two and doing routine chores is not a vacation either.

Is there anything else you would like to add?

High energy alone does not equate to success. Being energized, motivated, focused, balanced, and pacing yourself will bring you closer to your goals.

STEPHANIE DEL VALLE

Stephanie Del Valle
Certified Life Coach
718-931-0236
stephanie@personaljourneys.com
www.personaljourneys.com

Stephanie is a certified life coach and co-founder of Personal Journeys™. Her accreditation in life coaching is from the NLP and the Coaching Training Institute of California. Stephanie previously worked for Weight Watchers™—an eleven-year period that included staff training and development, one-on-one leader coaching, counseling of fellow staff members, and client counseling. As a corporate spokesperson for Weight Watchers, Stephanie has appeared on television programs such as *The Today Show, The Daily Show, NY1, WABC, and WNBC.* Additionally, she has been quoted in a number of magazines including *Vogue, New York Magazine, and Weight Watchers Magazine.* Stephanie has also done private counseling for Metro Diet and Dr. Barry Sears's Zone Cuisine.

Stephanie is remarkable. She has a passion for helping her clients love their bodies and themselves no matter what their weight is. Stephanie believes that once you can accept yourself, you are ready for real change regarding your health. She is a gifted person who is committed to her craft and to being an extraordinary coach. Her drive and love for life has been an inspiration to me.

Stephanie, is it possible to have a high amount of energy at work?

Absolutely. Feeling energetic is a result of making good choices.

What keeps people from feeling great at work every day?

Poor nutrition, not enough stress-reduction and rest, not enough regular physical activity, not believing that they can feel great at work every day, and having a negative mind-set.

If you are consistently tired at work, what is a healthy way to get more energy?

Breathe, stretch, change your body position, take a quick walk around the office, drink cold water, and if you are hungry, eat fruits, veggies, and nuts.

In addition, deal with whatever is weighing you down mentally. Figure out what is making you tired. Is it a specific task you need to get done that you've been postponing? Do that task first to feel the greatest relief. Or is it a larger, long-term worry or concern? If it is, decide on one step you can take to address it. One small step can lead to a solution. There is energy in action.

You are at your desk and you have three large projects to finish by 5:00 PM. You are hungry. You look over and see that your co-worker has a large bowl of candy sitting on her desk. What do you do?

When you're hungry, eat. But choose healthy foods. Healthy foods will make you less dependent on sugar to keep you going. Healthy foods are recognizable because they come from the land. There's no such thing as a potato chip bush.

What are some healthy foods?

Healthy foods include lean proteins like chicken breast, turkey breast, lean ground or trimmed beef, shellfish (shrimp, crab, lobster, clams, oysters, and mussels), eggs, low-fat cottage cheese, whey protein, and tofu.

Healthy vegetables include artichokes, broccoli, cabbage, cauliflower, celery, cucumbers, eggplant, garlic, ginger, green beans, leafy salad greens, mushrooms, okra, onions, peas, peppers, spinach, squash, tomatoes, and zucchini.

Healthy fruits include apples, apricots, avocados, berries, cantaloupes, cherries, figs, grapes, honeydew melon, kiwi, lemons, limes, nectarines, oranges, peaches, pears, plums, strawberries, and tangerines.

Healthy beans and legumes include black beans, chick peas, fava beans, kidney beans, lentils, lima beans, navy beans, peas, pinto beans, and soybeans.

Healthy grains include brown rice, wild rice, barley, whole oats, whole wheat, and whole-grain pastas.

Healthy fat sources include canola oil, flaxseed oil, extra-virgin olive oil, peanut oil, fats found in all fish, seeds, and pure butter in small amounts.

When in doubt, lean toward what's healthy. You'll be better nourished and will be replenishing your body better.

It's your boss's birthday. The department chips in and gets him a cake. Everyone is eating a piece, including your boss and some other people whom you would like to impress. The cake looks delicious. It's 3:00 PM, and you could use a boost to help you finish the day. What do you do?

Are you hungry? If not, don't eat the cake. Sip water, seltzer, or any non-caloric beverage instead. If you are hungry, decide how to balance the piece of cake against the rest of your day. Can you exercise after work, make lighter food choices later, or eat less tomorrow?

If you really want a piece, have a small slice and enjoy it. Taste and savor every bite. Then get back on track. Don't use the piece of cake as an excuse because you've "blown it." Focus on your victories and not your shortcomings.

You have a big presentation to give tomorrow. All you can think about is doing a good job. It's 6:00 PM, and you are still at your desk. What can you do to make sure that you are in the best possible mental and physical condition for tomorrow's presentation?

Do what athletes do before a crucial race: they visualize winning beforehand. See yourself successfully delivering your presentation. Make a movie in your mind of the good job you will do that's rich in every detail: the color, the sound, the framing, the emotion, the movement, etc. What do you hear? What do you see? Feel the feelings of success and victory. Play the movie over and over again until you are comfortable. Your presentation will go much more smoothly, because you've lived it successfully many times in your head.

In addition, be prepared. Get familiar with the setup of the presentation room. Eat well. Sleep well. Stretch and/or exercise. This will ensure that you feel well for your presentation.

You want to go to night school in order to advance your career. But your day job is stressful and demanding. What can you do to get the energy to do both?

Make sure that you're eating healthily and drinking plenty of water. This will provide the most nutritional support so that your energy level can be at its highest.

Also, strive to keep your core strong. Strong support in your body leads to strong support in your life. When your core is strong, the organs contained within your core (your heart, lungs, stomach, intestines) are well supported and therefore will function better. This makes your entire system and energy level stronger.

You want to start a healthy new phase in your life and career. What are some steps you can take? Where is the best place to begin?

Begin with the vision of where you want to be, and then decide that your future will contain the vision you have created. Determine what actions you will take to live the healthy life you've envisioned. Plot out a step-by-step plan linking those actions together, and start doing each step consistently. You will be on your way to living your healthy new life.

You have begun to eat better. You have even started an exercise program. Your boss walks into your office and tells you to pack your bags. You are going overseas. What can you do to make sure that you take your new healthy habits with you?

Look ahead at how you can pursue your healthy lifestyle at your destination. How long are you there for? If your stay is short-term, check out the hotel facilities beforehand to see how they can help you maintain your new healthy habits. Think about the cuisine of the country you're going to, and plan out what you will eat. Investigate available options for food—in-house restaurants, nearby restaurants, delivery options, nearby supermarkets, etc. And don't forget to hydrate with clean water.

If it's long-term trip, bring items with you, such as favorite snacks individually packaged (almonds, dried fruit, cereals, cans of tuna), exercise bands, DVDs, a mat, light hand-weights, sneakers, and music. Your goal is to make the best possible choices every chance you get. If you do, you can be successful.

What are some simple, practical, and easy-to-follow steps you can take to have more energy at work and feel great every day?

- Keep your exposure to energy-draining people to a minimum. Cultivate good relationships with positive, life-affirming, and forward-moving people.

- Focus your attention on the positive achievements and experiences you will have each day. Look forward to good things happening to you in your career.

- Plan your day to release stress from worry or concern. Get the big things done first for the boost that comes from accomplishing what matters most and makes the biggest difference. This burst of energy, whether psychic or physical, can propel you into your next task with zest, vigor, and a positively victorious mind-set.

- Hydrate regularly. Know where the bathroom is ahead of time.

- Choose the high road in all of the decisions you are faced with. Go with what feels right to you.

These steps will all lead to high energy and peace of mind.

What are some simple, practical, and easy-to-follow steps you can take to be healthier outside of work so that you can feel great and have more energy at your job every day?

- Prioritize what matters most in your personal life and focus your energy on those things first. You will get more accomplished in your life, which will leave you with more time and energy available for your job.

- Make sure to have downtime for yourself—at least fifteen minutes per day and longer if possible.

- Build body movement into your day-to-day lifestyle. Do active things with your family and friends. Walk and take the stairs whenever you can. Park farther away from the store than you normally would, and walk the rest of the way. Movement will give you energy and vitality. Plus, you will feel better.

What would you say to someone who says "I have no time" or "I have no energy" to implement the steps you've suggested?

People who say that they have no time or no energy are lying to themselves. They just don't want to change their circumstances at the moment.

If people had high energy, what would be possible for them in their careers?

Those that live the high-energy lifestyle have the potential to accomplish so much more than those with low to no energy. High-energy people often have a brighter outlook that has a positive effect on the way they see themselves, others, and their work. The vitality they feel extends to their approach to work and its challenges. They see themselves overcome challenges daily by finding ways to stay with their lifestyle choices. They do it because they see and feel the positive benefits of their efforts in how good they feel, look, and perform. Over time, those habits spill over into how they conduct their work-life, having the same positive effect.

People will be able to expand their vision and see more possibilities for themselves in most situations. They will be more likely to attempt more and will therefore achieve more. Much more of their potential will be realized, which is immensely positive for both them and their company.

What steps would you consider essential to a high-energy career success plan?

- Learning a healthy lifestyle with balanced eating and regular body movement.
- Focusing the mind on thinking positively.
- Having commitment to personal development.
- Planning and prioritizing.
- Taking time for meditation/self-time.
- Practicing stress-reduction and getting enough rest.
- Having reward systems in place.
- Having consistent and regular fun.

Is there anything else you would like to add?

Learn to enjoy *you*. You're the only person that you are guaranteed to have in your life from birth to death. Develop a great relationship with yourself based on respect, enjoyment, playfulness, and growth. If you do, you'll be set for life.

JEN BLACKERT

Jen Blackert
Business & Life Coach
12607 Silver Creek, Austin, TX 78727
512-671-3911
www.jenblackert.com

Jen Blackert has a BS in nutritional sciences from Virginia Tech, is a certified Pilates-method instructor, a certified yoga teacher, and a certified professional co-active coach. Jen spent thirteen years in corporate America, holding executive marketing positions at large global corporations.

Jen left the corporate grind and launched an online/telephone nutritional coaching business which she managed to fill with clients in eight months. Jen still coaches, but now focuses on helping businesses grow through marketing and attracting customers. The foundation of her practice is based on the laws of attraction and the power of thought and belief. I met Jen online and was so impressed with her background, philosophies, and outlook that I had to include her in this book.

Jen, is it possible to have a high amount of energy at work?

Absolutely. It's as simple as following an energy-balanced diet, getting regular exercise, living consciously, and listening to your body's energy needs.

What keeps people from feeling great at work every day?

They get overwhelmed and overstressed, and they stop listening to their bodies. This leads to emotional and mindless eating. Mindless behavior disrupts sleep patterns, states of being, and health.

You are at your desk and you have three large projects to finish by 5:00 PM. You are hungry. You look over and see that your co-worker has a large bowl of candy sitting on her desk. What do you do?

You stop. Take two or three breaths, and then choose the apple or cheese that you have stored in your desk drawer. When you are hungry, eat healthy foods. Sugar will raise your blood-sugar levels, intensify anxiety, cause cravings, and ensure that you will be hungry again very soon.

It's your boss's birthday. The department chips in and gets him a cake. Everyone is eating a piece, including your boss and some other people whom you would like to impress. The cake looks delicious. It's 3:00 PM, and you could use a boost to help you finish the day. What do you do?

It's important to participate in corporate activities and enjoy the pleasure of food on special occasions. You can have a piece the size of your palm. If you know there will be cake served later in the day, have a high-protein lunch, so that the effects of the sugar won't cause a strong impact on your blood sugar later.

You have a big presentation to give tomorrow. All you can think about is doing a good job. It's 6:00 PM, and you are still at your desk. What can you do to make sure that you are in the best possible mental and physical condition for tomorrow's presentation?

Inhale and exhale deeply about twenty times. Breathing calms the nervous system. Your big presentation won't seem as big anymore. Repeat as necessary.

You are tired. Your child was sick and kept you up all last night. You have a meeting with your boss in an hour. What can you do to get more energy for that meeting?

Do a few easy stretches. Twist around your chair and hold for five breaths. Then twist the other way. Cool water dabbed on your face is also great for puffiness and alertness, and can wake you up quickly.

You want to go to night school in order to advance your career. But your day job is stressful and demanding. What can you do to get the energy to do both?

This is a good time to do some work on where you see yourself in the future. Close your eyes and pretend you have a flashlight. The flashlight is focused on what you will gain by going to school. Search for the reason why you are going to school, and see yourself happily sitting in the classroom. Hold on to this reason and picture to motivate and energize you.

You want to start a healthy new phase in your life and career. What are some steps you can take? Where is the best place to begin?

The first step is your diet. Get it under control. When your diet is out of control, *you* are out of control. The next step is getting your mind-set in a good place by focusing on positive thinking and what you really want out of life. Lastly, incorporate exercises that work for your body and schedule.

You have begun to eat better. You have even started an exercise program. Your boss walks into your office and tells you to pack your bags. You are going overseas. What can you do to make sure that you take your healthy new habits with you?

Promise yourself that you will stick with your healthy new habits even while you are away. Write your promise down and read it every day. Where you are located doesn't matter—you can still eat healthily and exercise wherever you are.

What are some simple, practical, and easy-to-follow steps you can take to have more energy at work and feel great every day?

- Eat mindfully and consciously. Plan to have healthy snacks on hand for when you are hungry.
- Listen to your body. It knows what it needs and doesn't need.
- Reduce your stress level.
- Breathe deeply regularly to calm yourself.

What are some simple, practical, and easy-to-follow steps you can take to be healthier outside of work so you can feel great and have more energy at your job every day?

Have fun, play games, and give your mind time to be free from work.

What would you say to someone who says "I have no time" or "I have no energy" to implement the steps you've suggested?

I would tell them that they might want to reconsider these statements. Do they want to be well or not? If someone wants to be well, then they can make the time to be well. It's their decision. If you don't take care of yourself, no one else will take care of you. If you choose not to take care of yourself, your health will suffer.

What steps would you consider essential to a high-energy career success plan?

- Nurture and honor yourself with regular personal care, like massage, reiki, or pedicures.
- Give yourself energy with positive inner thoughts.
- Eat a balanced diet and take vitamins.
- Choose exercise that is fun, so that you will want to do it regularly.
- Incorporate spiritual practice into your life and routine.

HOLLY ANNE SHELOWITZ

Holly Anne Shelowitz
holly@nourishingwisdom.com
www.nourishingwisdom.com
845-687-9666

Holly is a board-certified nutrition counselor, whole-foods chef, and corporate health educator. She offers corporate workshops, classes, and nutrition programs. Holly also conducts long-distance cooking classes—she e-mails you a list of ingredients and supplies to buy, you call a special phone number at an appointed time, and you cook along with folks from all over the world.

I met Holly while researching this book, and I instantly loved and admired her philosophies and the difference she was making in the health of so many people. I asked Holly to participate in this book, and when she said yes, I was thrilled because I knew the book would be better because of her contribution.

Holly, is it possible to have a high amount of energy at work?

Yes.

What keeps people from feeling great at work every day?

In my practice, I notice that many people are sleep-deprived and removed from their body's natural rhythms. In addition, relying on coffee, sugar, or chocolate as regular sources of energy is hard on the body.

If you are consistently tired at work, what is a healthy way to get more energy?

Stretch, breathe, or take a quick walk around the block. This will help get your energy and heart moving. In addition, be sure to drink plenty of water. Often you will feel fuzzy-headed and drained when you are dehydrated.

You are at your desk and you have three large projects to finish by 5:00 PM. You are hungry. You look over and see that your co-worker has a large bowl of candy sitting on her desk. What do you do?

It's a great idea to keep some "real-food" snacks at your desk or in the refrigerator for moments like this—raw nuts, raisins, yogurt, fruit, cheese, cottage cheese, peanut or almond butter, and jam on crackers (this one also takes care of a desire for something sweet). Canned soups can also easily be heated up in the microwave.

It's your boss's birthday. The department chips in and gets him a cake. Everyone is eating a piece, including your boss and some other people whom you would like to impress. The cake looks delicious. It's 3:00 PM, and you could use a boost to help you finish the day. What do you do?

Deprivation can be stressful. Have a small piece, and let yourself enjoy it. Really taste it. In addition, you can accept a piece of cake and not eat the whole thing. Nobody has to know.

You have a big presentation to give tomorrow. All you can think about is doing a good job. It's 6:00 PM, and you are still at your desk. What can you do to make sure that you are in the best possible mental and physical condition for tomorrow's presentation?

Do your best to get a good night's sleep. Eat healthy foods for dinner—protein, lots of vegetables, and a small amount of carbs. Eat a great breakfast—a vegetable omelette, or a smoothie if you are too nervous to eat. Smoothies can be great breakfasts—put some yogurt and fruit into a blender with some whey protein powder, blend, and you are ready to go.

You are tired. Your child was sick and kept you up all last night. You have a meeting with your boss in an hour. What can you do to get more energy for that meeting?

Get fresh air or do some simple exercises at your desk, such as doing jumping jacks or skipping rope. This can be very energizing. Five minutes of movement can get your blood circulating and create natural energy.

You want to go to night school in order to advance your career. But your day job is stressful and demanding. What can you do to get the energy to do both?

See if it's possible to work a bit less, so that you are not time crunched. If you can't work less, be sure that your school schedule will not push you against the wall. Also, put time into meal planning, obtaining real-food snacks, and getting rest on weekends. You will want to incorporate good habits that will support your health.

You want to start a healthy new phase in your life and career. What are some steps you can take? Where is the best place to begin?

- Notice how you feel right now. What do you want to change? Why?
- If you are tired and have low ebbs of energy during the day, drink more water.
- Look at what you eat for breakfast. Are you eating a typical breakfast of sugary cereal, bagels, doughnuts, or just coffee? Try eating egg-whites or drinking a smoothie instead.
- Increase your vegetable consumption.
- Reduce white bread and pasta, and experiment with whole grains.
- Go to your local natural-food store, buy a few foods you haven't had before and learn ways to prepare them.
- Create a daily exercise routine. Even if you start doing simple stretches in the morning, it's better than nothing at all.
- Work with a health counselor or coach, or have a buddy—a friend or co-worker—to team up with. It can be difficult to make changes on your own.
- Go slow.

What would you say to someone who says "I have no time" or "I have no energy" to implement the steps you've suggested?

These two comments suggest why it's a perfect time to start. If they say they have no time, I would ask why they want to change, and ask them to focus on that instead. If they have no energy, I would say that this is their body's way of asking for help, and that a few small changes can make a big difference.

If people had high energy, what would be possible for them in their careers?

Honestly, anything they want.

What steps would you consider essential to a high-energy career success plan?

Eating foods that are truly nourishing (protein, lots of vegetables, fresh fruit), minimizing white flour and refined sugar, not rushing through meals, drinking water, having a daily exercise routine, and loving your work.

Is there anything that you would like to add?

Yes—eat with presence. Be aware of how certain foods make you feel. Listen to your body so that you can discover if it's better for you to eat at certain times of the day. Ask yourself if you sense a difference when you consume specific foods. If you aren't exercising, how is that affecting your energy level? Have you implemented routines like getting good sleep, eating greens, and practicing yoga? This is your body. Your goal is to look and feel your best.

THOMAS J. IANNIELLO

Dr. Thomas J. Ianniello, D.C.
North Isle Chiropractic
93 Miller Place Road, Miller Place, NY 11764
631-476-4051
www.northislechiropractic.com

Thomas is a licensed chiropractor, a graduate of New York Chiropractic College, a member of the Doctor's Speakers Bureau, and has been in private practice since 1993. He is also a student of functional medicine under the guidance of Dr. William G. Timmins. Dr. Timmins is the founder and program director at BioHealth Diagnostics. Tapping into functional medicine has allowed Thomas to treat patients at a much deeper level. He can assess and correct biochemical stress and/or infections in the body, in addition to treating situational stress through chiropractic care.

I met Thomas at a health fair. I sat through his informative seminar, filled out a questionnaire regarding my health, visited his office to have my results analyzed, and then hired him to help me get healthier.

Thomas has had a tremendous impact on my energy level and health. Through his easy, in-home testing, I was able to discover that my adrenaline system was burnt out, and that I had several stomach infections which were contributing to my constant bloating. Thomas was able to diagnose and discover why my energy level was low when no one else could figure it out. Furthermore, I was able to treat most of what was going wrong in my body without medication.

Thomas, is it possible to have a high amount of energy at work?

Yes, if your body is running properly.

What keeps people from feeling great at work every day?

When their bodies are not working efficiently. This leads to poor energy, poor mood, and poor production. When you rely on refined sugar and caffeine to give you energy, your body does not run very well. Your energy goes up and down. One moment you feel great, and shortly afterward you are crashing. In addition, job dissatisfaction raises your stress levels significantly.

If you are consistently tired at work, what is a healthy way to get more energy?

Eat a balanced meal including lots of pure water with protein and complex carbohydrates. Use the palm of your hand as a guide to the amount of protein to eat. Complex carbohydrates should be the size of your whole hand, with a thumbnail's worth of fat. Avoid refined sugar and caffeine, as the energy they create will only be temporary.

You are at your desk and you have three large projects to finish by 5:00 PM. You are hungry. You look over and see that your co-worker has a large bowl of candy sitting on her desk. What do you do?

Keep healthy snacks on hand, such as a protein bar, protein shake, an apple, or celery sticks. By being prepared with small meals and healthy snacks, you won't crave or need candy for energy.

It's your boss's birthday. The department chips in and gets him a cake. Everyone is eating a piece, including your boss and some other people whom you would like to impress. The cake looks delicious. It's 3:00 PM, and you could use a boost to help you finish the day. What do you do?

Now is not the right time to be "Superman," and resist the piece of cake. Eat a small piece—not so much for the burst of energy, but for the social grace of the situation. Being social at work is important. Being seen as the party-pooper might hurt your career.

You have a big presentation to give tomorrow. All you can think about is doing a good job. It's 6:00 PM, and you are still at your desk. What can you do to make sure that you are in the best possible mental and physical condition for tomorrow's presentation?

Finish your presentation material completely. Then review it slowly in a relaxed manner. Avoid an "all-nighter." Get a good night's sleep. Being fully rested will allow your brain to function better, and you will be sharper the next day.

You are tired. Your child was sick and kept you up all last night. You have a meeting with your boss in an hour. What can you do to get more energy for that meeting?

Make sure that you have eaten a good breakfast. A good choice is an egg-white omelette with broccoli, spinach, or some other type of dark green vegetable. This type of meal will give you a natural boost, meaning that you will burn the energy it provides at a consistent rate throughout the day.

You want to go to night school in order to advance your career. But your day job is stressful and demanding. What can you do to get the energy to do both?

Make sure you get eight hours of sleep every night, preferably from 10:00 PM to 6:00 AM. Your body heals between 10:00 PM and 2:00 AM, and your mind heals between 2:00 AM and 6:00 AM.

Also, eat balanced and healthy meals—six throughout the day, every two to three hours. Drink half your body weight (that is, in ounces) of water every day.

You want to start a healthy new phase in your life and career. What are some steps you can take? Where is the best place to begin?

The quickest and most effective action you can take is to cleanse your liver and kidneys through a detoxification program. This will remove toxicity from your organs and give you a clean slate to build from.

Remove all unnatural processed and packaged foods from your diet. These foods are addictive, have no nutritional value, and are empty, wasted calories. In addition, these foods put stress on your organs, increase your cholesterol level, and raise your blood pressure. Real food does not have a shelf life of more than a few days. Fresh organic fruits, vegetables, and meats will nourish your body and increase your energy level.

Make sure you enjoy your work. Having purpose in your career can drive your energy level up or down. Low purpose equals low energy. High purpose equals high energy.

You have begun to eat better. You have even started an exercise program. Your boss walks into your office and tells you to pack your

bags. You are going overseas. What can you do to make sure that you take your healthy new habits with you?

Drink predominantly bottled water on your trip to prevent parasite and bacterial infections. If you are preparing your own meals, wash all vegetables and fruits to remove pesticides. Stay away from raw or uncooked fish or meat as these are breeding grounds for parasites.

Avoid fast foods. If ordering from restaurants, request that your meat, chicken, or fish be baked or grilled. Stay away from bread, cereal, and pasta, as these foods will slow you down. Eat small healthy meals six times a day.

Exercise. The simplest form of exercise is walking. A good walk can clear your mind and put your cardiovascular system into fat-burning mode.

What would you say to someone who says "I have no time" or "I have no energy" to implement the steps you've suggested?

Tackle the most difficult task first. By confronting the toughest task and finishing it, the rest of your day will seem easier. Plus, you won't have to worry about this task anymore. Less mental energy wasted on worry means more energy available for other projects.

If you think about it, we all have the same amount of time—168 hours each week to work, play, and rest. Write out what you are doing with your time. Are you using it effectively, or wasting it because you are too tired or overworked?

To make real change, you have to make a firm, unyielding, conscious choice to change. Remember the last time you knew it was time to change something. Once you decided, no one could stop you, right? If you know what needs to be done, and you are not taking the steps necessary to improve your energy level, then you haven't really decided to change.

If people had high energy, what would be possible for them in their careers?

High energy would allow people to get work done more effectively than they ever envisioned. There is no project that cannot get done with the right energy behind it. High energy allows you to visualize your goals and then see them through to completion. In addition, physical energy drives the emotional and spiritual creativity that leads to success.

What steps would you consider essential to a high-energy career success plan?

- Eating only natural organic foods.
- Staying away from processed foods.
- Avoiding refined sugar and caffeine.
- Getting enough sleep at night.
- Reducing stress.
- Drinking water.
- Exercising.
- Changing habits that no longer serve you.
- Having emotional and spiritual energy.
- Achieving passion, intention, and purpose.
- Biochemistry maintenance and balance.

Is there anything else you would like to add?

If you are tired, it may mean that your adrenal system is burnt out. Get an evaluation of your adrenal system, along with other parts of your body, with simple at-home tests. For my patients, I use a laboratory that utilizes the highest clinical standards in testing and evaluation to ensure accurate results.

If you truly want high energy, keep an open mind and search for the best people for the treatment of your health. Quick fixes don't work. Health is earned, not given. It is not necessary to sacrifice your health to achieve success. Keep everything in balance—work, play, and rest—and success will follow. Put time into your health, and you'll achieve whatever you want.

Conclusion

This book has been a journey. My wish is that you have enjoyed it.

Did you learn a lot? I hope so. You were the reason I wrote this book.

No matter where you are today, high energy is waiting for you tomorrow. I was a person who had low energy, and now I'm not that person anymore. Who am I? A regular person just like you, who wanted to feel better.

If I can get my energy back, then so can you. Good luck to you.

Appendix A: Resources

Here are some resources that will help you get your energy back. If there is something that is inaccurate or should be added in a future edition, please send the correction or addition to: info@surpassyourdreams.com

Important Web Sites:

http://www.honestfoodguide.org
A free, downloadable public health and nutrition chart that dares to tell the truth about what foods we should really be eating

http://www.healingfoodreference.com
A free online reference database of healing foods, phytonutrients, and plant-based medicines that prevent or treat diseases and health conditions

http://www.naturalhealthlibrary.com
Offers more than fifteen free, downloadable books and interviews on natural health solutions

http://www.herbreference.com
A free online reference library that lists medicinal herbs and their health benefits

http://www.diseaseproof.com
A forum that promotes discussion on health information to help people understand how to take control of their health through nutritional excellence

http://www.obesity.org
A leading organization for advocacy and education regarding obesity

Informative Articles and Where to Find Them:

"Ways to Improve Your Health"
http://www.nourishingwisdom.com/articles/twelve-ways.html

"Tips for Eating While You Work"
http://beactiveyork.com/beactiveyork/content/dianework.aspx

"Having Lunch at Your Desk—Again? Here's How to Make it Healthier"
http://onhealth.webmd.com/script/main/art.asp?articlekey=60828

"Diet Wreckers in Your Desk"
http://www.prevention.com/article/0,5778,s1-4-57-190-4817-1-P,00.html

"Healthy Food/Snack Choices"
http://www.ccohs.ca/healthyworkplaces/topics/healthyeating.html

"Ways to Nourish Yourself"
http://www.nourishingwisdom.
com/articles/seven-ways-to-nourish-yourself.html

"Food Traps and What You Can Do About Them"
http://www.lifetimefitness.com/magazine/index.
cfm?strWebAction=article_detail&intArticleId=509

"Tips for Nourishing Yourself at Work—Without Eating a Thing"
http://www.nourishingwisdom.com/articles/seven-ways-to-nourish-your-self.html

"Causes of Obesity Other Than Over-Eating"
http://www.foxnews.com/story/0,2933,201397,00.html

"Too Big to Work? Obesity Screening Called Unfair"
http://www.imdiversity.com/Villages/Careers/articles/
pns_obesity_discrimination_1204.asp

"Why Should a Workplace Be Concerned About Healthy Eating?"
http://www.ccohs.ca/healthyworkplaces/topics/healthyeating.html

"Promoting Healthy Eating at Work" http://www.wellnessinstitute.mb.ca/news/
articles/healthyeating_040505.php

"Too Busy to Exercise? Now You Can Work Out at Work"
http://exercise.about.com/cs/fittingitin/a/officeexercise.htm

"Exercise for the Deskbound: Take a Short Break from Your Routine to Relieve Some of the Back Pressures You May Feel While Sitting at Your Desk All Day"
http://www.findarticles.com/p/articles/mi_m1189/is_n6_v270/ai_21279892

"Exercise May Make You a Better Worker"
http://www.msnbc.msn.com/id/8160459/

"Managing Stress with Regular Exercise"
http://www.mindtools.com/stress/Defenses/Exercise.htm

"Workaholics Quiz: Do You Focus on Work Too Much?"
http://www.quintcareers.com/workaholics_quiz.html

"Tips for Reducing Workaholism"
http://www.quintcareers.com/workaholic.html

"Are Top Leaders Battling to Build Energy?"
http://www.clomedia.com/content/templates/clo_article.asp?articleid=425&zoneid=101

"Tips for When You Feel Tired"
http://www.healthatoz.com/healthatoz/Atoz/dc/cen/ment/sled/alert04132000.jsp

"The Value of Sleep"
http://ezinearticles.com/?The-Value-Of-Sleep&id=244170

"Snoozing at Work"
http://www.healthatoz.com/healthatoz/Atoz/dc/cen/ment/sled/alert04132000.jsp

"Tips for Making Sure Your Next Job Is the Right Job for You" http://www.6figurejobs.com/ExecNewsletter.cfm?CFID=3925897&CFTO-KEN=43680974&noCache=412801&NewsID=204&am=1#two

Note: To register for *free* access to a special web page that contains additional resources in addition to what's listed in this section, please visit:
http://www.surpassyourdreans.com/energyresources.html

Once you register, you will be notified of exclusive groups and classes that I will be conducting by telephone on this topic, as well as informed of important resource updates. You also will be able to simply click on the links found in this section, rather than having to type them into your browser. I hope you take advantage of this special resource, which I have created just for you.

About The Author

Deborah Brown-Volkman, credentialed coach and career expert.

Deborah Brown-Volkman is a professional certified coach (PCC) and the president of Surpass Your Dreams, Inc.—a successful career, life, and mentor coaching company that has been delivering a message of motivation, success, and personal fulfillment since 1998. She specializes in four areas:

1. Career coaching for senior executives, vice presidents, and managers who are looking for new career opportunities or seek to become more productive in their current role.

2. Life coaching for those who want to improve other areas of their lives in addition to their career.

3. Start-up and practice-building for those who want to make coaching their next career.

4. Marketing, public relations, and writing services for those who want recognition and fame in their career.

Current and former clients include individuals from: JPMorganChase, Oracle Corporation, Lucent Technologies, General Motors, Procter & Gamble, Ziff Davis, IBM, American Express, EDS, Ogilvy & Mather, McCann-Erickson Worldgroup, Columbia University, New York University, Chief Executive Magazine, MSNBC, and BMW.

Deborah Brown-Volkman is a published writer, and her articles on how to be successful in your career can be found on hundreds of web-sites. She is the author of three books: *Coach Yourself To A New Career (A Guide for Discovering Your Ultimate Profession)*, *Four Steps to Building a Profitable Coaching Practice (A Complete Marketing Resource Book for Coaches)* and *Four Steps to Building a Profitable Business (A Marketing Start-Up Guide for Business Owners, Entrepreneurs, and Professionals)*, and co-author of *The Essential Coaching Book (Secrets to a Winning Life from the Professional and Personal Coaches of the United*

Coaching Associates, Inc.). Deborah Brown-Volkman also writes an e-mail newsletter titled *Surpass Your Dreams,* which offers you practical advice and steps to make Monday the best day of your work-week.

Deborah Brown-Volkman has been featured as a career expert for WABC-TV's *New York Eyewitness News,* CNN, News 12, *The Wall Street Journal, The New York Times, Smart Money Magazine, Business 2.0, The Chicago Tribune, and New York Newsday.* She was also a featured guest on BBC Radio Scotland when they came to New York City to find out how people were coping in their careers since the September 11th attacks.

Deborah Brown-Volkman is a graduate of Coach University's Coaches Program, enrolled in CoachVille's Graduate School of Coaching, an International Coach Federation (ICF) professional certified coach (PCC), and a 2004 recipient of CoachVille's Annual Thomas Leonard coaching award for contributing to the success and evolution of coaching. She is a founding member of Coachville.com, a coaching-training portal created by the founder of Coach University; a member of the International Association of Coaches, New York City Midtown Coaching Center, and 24/7 Coach; a member of the International Coach Federation (ICF), the most well-known and respected coaching organization in the world; a member of the Moriches Chamber of Commerce, Westhampton Chamber of Commerce, and Moriches Rotary of New York; a career expert for LongIsland.com; and a charter member of the ICF-New York City Speakers Bureau.

Before becoming a coach, Deborah Brown-Volkman's background included twelve years running sales and marketing programs for Fortune 500 companies and dot-coms. She received an AAS degree in data processing from Queensborough Community College, a BBA in marketing from Hofstra University, and a certificate in financial planning from New York University.

Deborah Brown-Volkman lives with her husband and best friend Brian in Long Island, NY.

Deborah Brown-Volkman can be reached at info@surpassyourdreams.com or via her web site at http://www.surpassyourdreams.com

Endnotes

1. *Personnel Today* is the HR profession's news magazine in the UK. It is the first and only weekly publication serving the human resources market. Published every Tuesday, it is delivered to the workplaces of more than 50,000 HR and training professionals. URL for the article: http://www.personneltoday.com/Articles/2005/10/25/32213/Fattism+is+the+last+bastion+of+employee+discrimination.htm

2. Pfizer Inc. study published in the *Journal of Occupational and Environmental Medicine*. URL of report: http://www.news-medical.net/?id=6816

3. FOX 13 in Tampa Bay, Florida. Segment ran on November 4, 2005. URL for segment: http://www.wtvt.com/info/nycu11-05.html

4. Excerpt taken from an article titled: "Diet Wreckers in Your Desk" written by Karen Cicero for prevention.com. URL of article: http://www.prevention.com/article/0,5778,s1-4-57-190-4817-1-P,00.html

5. URL for article: http://www.ezinearticles.com/?Sugar-Lovers-Beware&id=9389 Rino Soriano's web site is http://healthevolutioninternational.com

6. URL for article: http://www.advancingwomen.com/coffee/39585.php Emily Clark's web sites are at http://www.lifestyle-health-news.com & http://www.medical-health-news.com

7. URL for article: http://www.epigee.org/fitness/deal_with_carbs.html

8. URL for article: http://mentalhelp.net/poc/view_doc.php?type=doc&id=5915&cn=219 Updated July 11, 2005

9. URL for article: http://www.sixwise.com/newsletters/05/10/19/all_the_health_risks_of_processed_foods_—_in_just_a_few_quick_convenient_bites.htm Article is from and reprinted with permission from the free Security/Wellness e-Newsletter at SixWise.com

10. URL   of   article: http://www.whfoods.com/genpage.php?tname=george&dbid=107 The article was updated on July 11, 2005

11. URL of article: http://familydoctor.org/784.xml

12. URL source: http://www.metrokc.gov/dchs/mhd/mhm/quiz.htm Department of Community and Human Services in Seattle, WA

13. URL of article: http://www.athealth.com/Consumer/disorders/workstress.html

14. URL of article: http://boston.bizjournals.com/boston/stories/2003/07/14/smallb2.html?t=printable

15. URL of article: http://www.annecollins.com/diet-news/physical-activity.htm

16. URL of article: http://www.seniorjournal.com/NEWS/Fitness/2-12-09PhysicalActivity.htm

17. Reported by CNN on December 4, 2000. URL for article: http://archives.cnn.com/2000/CAREER/trends/12/04/napping/

18. URL sources: http://www.sleepfoundation.org & http://archives.cnn.com/2000/CAREER/trends/12/04/napping/

19. URL of article: http://www.quintcareers.com/workaholic.html

20. URL of article: http://www.fastcompany.com/articles/archive/workaholics.html Book was published by Bantam Books, 1995

21. URL of article: http://www.personneltoday.com/30836.articlev

22. URL for article: http://www.tec.net.au/index.php?itemID=165&branch=112

23. URL for article: http://www.6figurejobs.com/ExecNewsletter.cfm?CFID=2207177&CFTOKEN=36179556&noCache=982271&NewsID=46&am=1#one

24. URL for article: <u>http://www.columbuswired.</u>
    <u>net/Columns/SurpassYourDreams/</u>
    <u>AreYouInTheWrongCareer_011402.htm</u>

978-0-595-41263-1
0-595-41263-7

Printed in the United States
87067LV00004BA/288/A